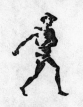

How to Eat Like a Thin Person

The Dieter's Handbook of Do's and Don'ts

Lorraine Dusky and J. J. Leedy, M.D.

Illustrations by Loretta Trezzo

Simon and Schuster   New York

Contents

Introduction

Are you overweight now and do you want to be slim? So you simply want to lose—and keep off—10 or 20 pounds? Have you always been fat but longed to be thin? Does your weight go up one month and down the next, only to go back up again? Would you like to put all that behind you?

We all know slimming down isn't that difficult to understand or explain: You eat less and exercise more and you lose weight. One, two, three, just like that. But it's in the doing that we fall down. Or we go on a diet for a few weeks, maybe even months, and the weight falls off just as it's supposed to, but it returns when we go back to our old eating habits.

What most of us don't realize is that to be slim and stay that way—if you have a tendency to weigh more than you would like—requires that you make major changes in your life. You will consistently have to consume fewer calories than when you were heavy; regular exercise—something you enjoy doing enough to keep on doing it—must be a part of your day-to-day routine. It's like being a reformed alcoholic; you have to be aware of your problem day in, day out, year after year. If you let up, you'll gain back that weight.

Not surprisingly, a recent study at the University of California found that people who lose weight with the help of such techniques as keeping a record of what they eat, weighing themselves regularly, and exercising frequently are more likely to keep the weight off if they *keep doing these same things periodically*.

And whenever we read an interview with a famous model about how she stays so slim, her answer invariably begins something like this: "I weigh myself first thing in the morning. . . ." What she means is that she reminds herself every single day that she must at least be aware of what she eats, and she uses the best piece of biofeedback equipment available to all of us—the bathroom scale. You lose a pound and you get immediate gratification; you gain a pound, you know right away it's time to cut back.

While to stay slim you will have to be on daily watch, life ahead doesn't have to be a dismal succession of days without an occasional piece of chocolate cake or slice of Sicilian pizza. If you deny yourself something that you really love—and see no time in the future when you can ever have it again—you are likely to feel defeated at the start and give up immediately. What we will help you do is choose to have that something special more *then* than *now*. And in time, this new eating behavior, just like anything else, will not seem so foreign or tedious, but easy, the way things are supposed to be.

Remember the first time you drove a car? You undoubtedly veered all over the place and jammed on the brakes when you meant to come to a slow stop. Eventually, driving became nearly as simple as walking. You learned a new behavior and made it a part of your life. That's what this book will help you to do—make eating and thinking like a slim person seem normal. In time, you will learn to appreciate the taste of vegetables that have not been smothered in butter and rich sauces; an apple will seem like a better snack than a brownie; a gorgeous salad, with its combination of colors and textures, will be more appealing than greasy ribs. No, we are not crazy; we are only saying that you can learn to change your eating preferences so that the meal of choice is what a thin person would select. You will have learned how to eat like a thin person.

This book contains no specific diet. It works with any diet you choose. Oh, there are food and nutrition tips, but they are presented as guidelines to help you find an eating pattern that works for you and a way of living that is good enough for a lifetime. We'll tell you why exercise is so critical to a lean and healthy life, and we'll give you specific pointers on what various exercises do for you. We'll tell you how to incorporate more activity into your life so that in just living you burn off more calories than before. We'll give you mind games that will make sticking to your new diet plan easier. We'll tell you how to deal with your parents when you go to visit them and what to say to Aunt Clara when she proffers her famous cheesecake and expects you to eat half of it as you did when you were a kid. We'll help you deal with friends and relations who say they will be offended if you don't eat more; we'll tell you how to order in a restaurant and how to go to a cocktail party without turning it into an excuse for a binge. We'll help you keep that weight off once you've lost it and help you suggest how you can turn the people close to you into your allies against fat. And we'll help you deal with the new willowy you.

The book is arranged in sections so that you can flip to whatever you need quickly, when, say, you feel a snack attack coming on, or are about to face dinner at the boss's house. So let's get started. Why put off until tomorrow what you could lose today? Tomorrow you could already be one day into your new thin life.

1 Are You Overweight?

or, Is Your Scale Sending Out an SOS?

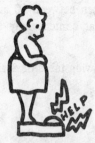

Now you probably don't need anyone to tell you that you are overweight. Your clothes may not fit the way you want them to—or you may be several sizes from your ideal figure. A bulge around the middle, thighs that are much more than they used to be, "love handles" at the sides of your waist and the hard, cold facts on the scale may give you more clues than you want. Yet for those who like to measure themselves against a specific ideal, here are several tests to try.

• Does your height minus your waist (in inches) equal more than 36? If so, you're in trouble. For a small frame, use 40 as the number to attain.

• For women, multiply your height in inches by 3.5 and then subtract 110. Thus a woman of five foot four (64 inches) should weigh about 114 pounds. For men, multiply your height by 4 and subtract 130. A six-foot male should therefore weigh approximately 158 pounds. Remember, these ideals do not take many factors into account—such as your amount of muscles and body frame—and they should only be viewed as approximate figures.

Are You Overweight?

• Two people who weigh the same and have similar body types may still have a large difference in their amount of fat tissue. That's why one woman at 125 may look thin, while the person sitting next to her who's the same height may look like a cream puff. One way to measure body fat is to take a fold of skin under your arm and pull it away from the muscle. Squeeze gently. If the amount of the fold is greater than one inch, you probably have a relatively high fat content. Between a half inch and an inch means you still have room to reduce. Below a half inch is normal, especially for men; women may have a bit more. This simple test works because more than half of our body fat is stored just beneath the skin. Normal healthy men are often between 10 and 13 percent fat, while the average woman's fat content may be as much as 25 percent.

• And, finally, we have included the following table of desirable weights.

Desirable Weights

Weight in Pounds According to Frame (In Indoor Clothing)

Men of Ages 25 and Over

HEIGHT (with shoes on) 1-inch heels		SMALL FRAME	MEDIUM FRAME	LARGE FRAME
Feet	Inches			
5	2	114-125	123-134	131-145
5	3	118-127	126-138	134-149
5	4	122-130	129-141	137-153
5	5	126-134	132-144	140-157
5	6	129-138	135-148	143-161
5	7	133-142	139-152	148-166
5	8	137-146	143-157	152-171
5	9	141-150	147-161	156-175
5	10	145-155	151-165	160-179
5	11	149-159	155-170	164-184
6	0	153-163	159-175	169-191
6	1	157-168	163-180	173-194
6	2	161-172	168-185	178-199
6	3	165-176	172-190	182-204
6	4	169-180	179-195	187-209

Women of Ages 25 and Over

HEIGHT (with shoes on) 2-inch heels		SMALL FRAME	MEDIUM FRAME	LARGE FRAME
Feet	Inches			
4	10	94-101	98-110	106-122
4	11	96-104	101-113	109-125
5	0	99-107	104-116	112-128
5	1	102-110	107-119	115-131
5	2	105-113	110-122	118-134
5	3	108-116	113-126	121-138
5	4	111-119	116-130	125-142
5	5	114-123	120-135	129-146
5	6	118-127	124-139	133-150
5	7	122-131	128-143	137-154
5	8	126-135	132-147	141-158
5	9	130-140	136-151	145-163
5	10	134-145	140-155	149-168
5.	11	138-152	144-159	153-173
6	0	140-155	149-162	158-175

2 The Commitment

or, Do You Really Want to Lose Weight?

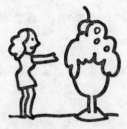

The question is a bit more complicated than it appears. Of course you want to lose weight, you are probably thinking—why else would I have picked up this book? But we are going to ask you to change your life—not simply go on a diet for a week or a month—and so the question is not so ridiculous. Do you really want to lose weight? Here are a few questions to consider:

• *Who wants you to lose weight?* Do you? Or is it someone else? Your mother, brother, sister, doctor, spouse, employer? Until you make the decision that you—and you alone—want to lose weight, taking off pounds will be nearly impossible. You'll think "Why shouldn't I have that Danish—I don't need to have anyone tell me what to do."

• *What will you gain if you lose weight?* Make a list. Include everything that comes to mind, no matter how trivial. You will not have trouble squeezing into theater or airline seats. You will not have trouble with seat belts. You will not be embarrassed when you have to squeeze through narrow openings. It will be a joy to get on the scale. Your love life may improve. You can shop for clothes anyplace you please. You can wear different styles and colors.

● *Do you think you will be happier?* Think this one over carefully. Perhaps you are not so unhappy now; yet it is true that low self-esteem and being overweight often go hand in hand. Once you lose the weight, you are likely to gain not only confidence, but the feeling that you can take charge in other areas of your life as well.

● *Will your health improve?* Slim people live longer, can expect fewer problems with the heart and lungs, and have a reduced risk of diabetes and several types of cancer.

● *Will you have greater career opportunities?* It's likely. One study found that 35 percent of the executives in the $10,000 to $20,000 salary range were at least 10 pounds overweight, while among those earning between $25–$35,000, only 10 percent were overweight. And remember, the cutoff point was a lousy 10 pounds. Another study found that an obese woman has one-third the chance of a normal woman of getting into a prestige college, the school of her choice, or any college at all. Whether it's because of the interviewer's unconscious discrimination or the low self-esteem of the overweight applicant is unclear. You might not like it, but there it is.

● *Are you thinking—but it will take too long?* Remember that time is going to pass anyway. Six months will be here when six months have passed, and either you will be thinner than you are right now or not. Time is going to pass no matter what you do. Remind yourself how quickly the future arrives. Wasn't it only yesterday that it was summer, or last year, or your seventeenth birthday? The future seems far away until it arrives.

There was a story in the newspaper about a young woman who climbed a mountain all by herself. At first, the task seemed impossible. It would take several weeks. How did she keep going, the reporters asked. "I kept asking myself—how do you eat an elephant?" she replied. "One bite at a time."

3 Are You a Compulsive Eater?

or, Do You Fantasize about Food When You're Making Love?

Test yourself. There's no one watching.

• Do you crave food at a certain time of the day—or night—that has nothing to do with mealtime?

• Do you always maintain that you can diet "when you want to" despite evidence to the contrary?

• Do you have feelings of guilt and remorse after overeating?

• Do you often eat when you are not hungry, but just because "it's something to do"?

• Do you look forward to the times and places when you can eat alone, secretly?

• Do you go on binges for no apparent reason?

- Do you plan these binges ahead of time?

- Do you eat to forget about worries and anxieties?

- Does your food obsession make you or others unhappy?

- Have you ever been treated by a doctor for being overweight?

- Do you eat sensibly in front of others and pig out when alone?

- Is your weight affecting the way you live?

- Are you afraid of what might happen if you lose weight?

If you answer yes to more than three questions, you probably are an eater who some time ago went on "automatic" feeding and whose eating habits bear little or no relationship to hunger and nutritional needs. It's time to change that. Only you can regain control of your life. We are not selling snake oil; we will simply help you nudge yourself into exercising your willpower, even though right now it seems buried.

4 Weight-Loss Research

or, There Ain't No Magic Bullet Yet

Since there are between 60 and 80 million fat people in this country, it is not all that hard to understand why, as a nation, we seem to be obsessed with weight. The average male is 18 pounds overweight; the average female is 21 pounds too heavy. Wouldn't it be wonderful if we could all just take some kind of pill that would make the fat melt away, right before our eyes, overnight? Well, there may be some such miracle in the future that will at least speed up the process.

A fatlike substance that can be substituted for shortening, used as a spread instead of butter, replace salad oil and the fat in ice cream and candy—and all without adding a single calorie—is being tested at various research centers around the country. Sucrose polyster (SPE) may cut the absorption of dietary cholesterol in the body *by half*. It dissolves the cholesterol in the intestines and carries it out of the body. Its main drawback is that it interferes with the absorption of vitamins A and E, but the researchers say that taking supplements avoids any problem.

When will it be available? FDA approval may be forthcoming in a year or two. However, it must be noted that current preparations that decrease the amount of dietary cholesterol absorbed, such as cholestyramine, taste terrible and must be ingested in large quantities. So although the research is encouraging, the results are not yet ideal.

A Harvard scientist reports that some overweight people have a lower level of an enzyme called adenosine triphosphatase (ATPase), which is responsible for between 10 to 50 percent of the body's production of heat and naturally helps our bodies burn off calories. On the average, fat people have 22 percent less ATPase than individuals of normal weight. The solution: Find a chemical that can turn ATPase on or off. Some people are looking, but don't count on it too soon.

Although you still have to learn to regulate how much you eat, a source of protein—more concentrated than soybeans or raw meat—may help you control those binges that are triggered by a drop in blood sugar. Spirulina, made from vegetable plankton, is 65 percent protein and contains phenylalanine, an amino acid that is believed to act directly on the hypothalamus. In effect, the algae informs the brain that it is getting the necessary fuel. The high-quality protein is easy to digest and thus is absorbed faster by the body than most proteins.

Several weight-loss specialists around the country are recommending spirulina to their patients, who are achieving dramatic results—but only if they are already motivated to lose weight. Spirulina grows in the fresh-water lakes of Africa and Central America where the natives have been eating it for centuries. It's available at health-food and vitamin stores in 500-milligram tablets or powdered form.

But leave those regular diet pills that promise to suppress appetite at the checkout counter. Hunger suppressants work for a few weeks before losing their effectiveness, when larger and larger doses are required. Side effects: nervousness and irritability, and if you are losing quickly, you are going to have to combat them anyway. And don't discount the possibility of a rebound weight gain once you go off the pills.

5 Keeping Track of What You Eat

or, Filling Out Your Food Forms

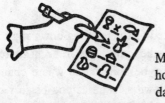 Most of us are not really aware of how much food we consume every day. You may think of yourself as a three-meals-a-day person, but really eat six times—if it's got calories, it counts. It doesn't matter if it's "only a cookie or two" with the midmorning coffee; it doesn't matter if it's "just a few beers" every night; it doesn't matter if it's a slice of pizza when shopping. Some people consume more calories "when it doesn't count" than they actually do at meals.

The best way to find out exactly what you are eating—and when and why—is to keep an accurate record of everything that goes into your mouth over a period of a week or two. This will let you analyze why you are overweight. Include everything but water, black coffee, or plain tea. Record the time you eat and where. Note if some specific event triggers the eating. Write down if you were alone or with others. Who? Were you doing anything else at the time—reading, talking on the telephone, watching television? Were you bored, depressed, or happy? Remember, it's okay to put down everything. You don't have to share this record with anyone.

• Buy yourself *two* calorie counters at your local bookstore. Select one that will suit your needs. You might take a sample menu or a list of some favorite foods with you and check to make sure they are included. Look for one with food measurements that make sense to you. Four ounces may be more accurate than a half cup, but only if you weigh everything. Try to find one that includes some brand-name items. You buy two so that you can carry one with you. After a while, the approximate caloric values of food will become second nature, and you will not need to resort to it every time you pick up an orange.

• Get a new notebook for the project, one that can be carried with you. Take it with you everywhere. It will serve as a reminder that everything you put into your mouth that has a single calorie must be recorded.

• Although you will be tempted to start cutting down right from the beginning, try not to. Only when you have an accurate record of your eating behavior will you be able to see where change is called for. If you start cutting down as soon as you begin recording, you will not learn what made all the calories add up in the first place. And you might fool yourself into thinking that you really don't eat much—it's heredity, or biochemical, or one of the million excuses that you can dream up.

• If you find that you are resisting record keeping, ask yourself why. It may be that you really do not want to lose weight at this time.

• Don't fool yourself into thinking that you can remember what you ate. You won't. And don't kid yourself by saying that you don't want to keep track because someone will see you and think you're foolish. If you must, make up an excuse, such as the fact that your doctor suspects an allergy, and he asked you to keep the records. And if you are truthful, most people will respect your seriousness and you, too—for finally doing something about your weight.

• Don't turn the records into a diary of guilt. Don't admonish yourself every time you write something in the diary. Accept the fact that you have been eating like this for quite some time, and tell yourself that you are doing this to better understand yourself and your behavior.

• If you continue to have trouble keeping the records, ask yourself exactly how much trouble is it? How long does it take each day? Fifteen minutes? Ten? Is that too much trouble when what you want to do is establish a new, sensible way of eating for life? Remember that we all resist change, and any new behavior feels awkward at first—tying your shoes, walking, riding a bicycle. All of these behaviors were once beyond your ability, but with practice, came to seem natural, easy. Keeping a record of what you eat is the only sure way of figuring out what you eat and why. It can be your most valuable aid to change.

Sample Food Diary

Breakfast	Calories	Alone or with Someone
Orange juice, 4 ounces	55	
Cooked cereal with ½ sliced banana and ½ cup milk	242	
Coffee, cream and sugar	47	
Midmorning snack		
Prune danish, huge	400	
Lunch		
Tuna salad sandwich on whole-grain bread	300	With Martha
Mixed green salad with lemon juice	30	from the
Baked custard—½ cup	150	office
Coffee with cream and sugar	47	
Snack		
Apple	80	
8 almonds	60	

Dinner

1 large loin lamb chop, broiled	355
½ cup cooked carrots	25
Medium-large baked potato	145
1 tablespoon sour cream for potato	25
½ cup green beans	15
¾ cup cole slaw with mayonnaise	85
Glass of red wine	100

10 P.M.

1 cup rich ice cream	330

Total	2491

Time Ate—Beginning and End	Where?	What Else Was Going On?	How Did I Feel?
1:15 to 2:00	Coffee Shop	Talking about her mother's diet and my husband's affair	Depressed, anxious

Analyzing Your Records

The food diary can turn out to be quite a revelation. Suppose you fix meals for your children that are separate from the rest of the family's. You may discover that you actually do so much "snacking" or "just tasting" during this period, that you are consuming the equivalent of a light lunch. You may discover that you are drinking more alcohol than you assumed. And many of you may discover that you are eating not because you are hungry, but because you are bored, depressed, or both. For a great many people, time on their hands means food in their mouths.

• How much time are you spending eating? Do you eat your meals in less than twenty or thirty minutes? Do you finish before others because you put another bite into your mouth before you have swallowed the last one? If you hurry the meal, not only are you hardly aware of what you are eating, you are not giving your body time to adjust to feeling full and telling you when to stop. You're too busy shoveling in the mounds to notice, and you're not letting food be the sensual pleasure it can be.

• Where are you eating? If you find that your records show you eat not only at the table, but in front of the TV, in bed, at the refrigerator while you decide what to eat for lunch, at your desk at work, while shopping—the list could go on, but you get the idea. For some people, nearly every room in the house provides a food cue of one sort or another. When you read in bed before retiring, do you always have a snack? Do you always have a drink or two while watching the news? These patterns may be so ingrained that you are hardly aware of what you are putting into your mouth. Select one place where you will eat all your meals while at home. Eat there and there alone. Yes, it will seem odd the first time you don't have milk and cookies along with your novel, but you expected that, didn't you? Remember: Unlearning any behavior and replacing it with another always seems awkward at first.

• At least for a while—and this is hardest if you live alone—don't do anything else while you are eating. Pay attention to the colors and textures of the food instead of something that distracts your attention from your meal. You are less likely to keep on eating and not notice that you are actually full. Notice the green of the spinach, the rosiness of a radish or two, the flaky texture of a baked potato. Savor each bit as if it were a rare treat. In fact, it may be one for you, if you have been wolfing down food for years without paying any attention to taste, color, texture. Sure, you will feel silly at first—all that fuss over a potato? But in time it won't seem silly at all. You'll wonder why you let yourself miss the real pleasure of dining.

• Note how you felt when you ate, especially the snacks. If you seem bored, or lonely, or tired, or depressed, you are using food to gratify a need that is best satisfied another way. After a half dozen chocolate chip cookies you are still bored, and now depressed because you've just eaten so much. We can't tell you how to get rid of those negative feelings for good, but there are some practical things you could do. If you're lonely, for instance, why not call a friend—or someone who's shut in and would be cheered by your call? You don't have to say why you're calling. Bored? There must be something you enjoy doing—or have always wanted to do. Now is the best time to begin. Learn how to knit. Plant a garden. Start a bird-feeding station and notice how many different types of birds visit. Take up that sport you always thought you'd enjoy. Not only will you have less time to eat, but the increased activity will burn up calories.

• Food, especially chocolate because of its chemical makeup, can lift your spirits but the mood elevation lasts only a short time and keeps you constantly behind the eight ball with your weight. Remember, to lose weight and keep it off, you must change the way you live.

• If you find you eat when you are angry—why take it out on yourself? No matter how difficult, summon up the courage to face the person who is making you mad and let him or her know. You don't necessarily have to go in yelling and screaming, but you can think through how to calmly tell that person what is upsetting you. Does your boss ask you to shop for his wife, and does it make you so angry that while shopping you stop and have a hot fudge sundae? Okay, you have treated yourself to fifteen minutes of company time, but your work is still there waiting. All you have done is punish yourself. The next time the boss asks you to shop or do something you don't like and, strictly speaking, isn't a part of your job, agree to do it, but say you would *prefer*—as tactfully as possible naturally—not to do it in the future.

• Or let's say your secretary has the annoying habit of eating her lunch at her desk and leaving the papers and crumbs on the desk top for the afternoon. It gives a messy impression of your office.

Instead of muttering to yourself and consoling yourself with cookies, ask your coworker to clean up after lunch.

• Perhaps it's something at home that bugs you. Your spouse doesn't put the cap back on the toothpaste. Or leaves the soap covered with dirty bubbles. Or leaves underwear on the floor all the time. Speak up rather than eat.

• If you can't express your anger directly to the person, think about what you would like to say—and punch a pillow or engage in some other physical activity.

• If you note that you are eating when you are tired, do something about the fatigue instead of making your digestive system work harder processing those extra calories. Take a nap. Take a relaxing bath or shower. Go for a walk.

• If your records show that you always eat something with a particular person, arm yourself in advance the next time the two of you are going to be together. Say to yourself: "No thanks, I think I'll skip the cupcake (or whatever) today." Be prepared for the other person's alarm—after all, most fatties like to have partners in crime. Practice in your mind how you will resist. It will make dealing with the situation much easier.

• Or you can try to restrict your visits with people who always put food in your path. Try meeting them elsewhere. If you usually meet someone in a coffee shop and order cake and coffee, suggest you meet in a park or at a street corner. Why not visit while taking a walk?

• Throughout the process of learning how to behave like a thin person, keeping a food diary can be the most important single thing you can do to stay motivated. Without the diary you may think that your midmorning snacks are not important. They only add up to 300 calories a day. For one day, it doesn't seem like much, but if you snack every morning for a year, you may gain more than 25 pounds!

The diary will help you analyze not only what you eat, but the situations and people who trigger eating. Once you know what the problem is, you can attack. Any general knows that you have to locate the enemy before the battle can begin. Think of yourself as the commander in chief waging a war against Personal Enemy No. 1: FAT. And now that you know where he is, you can begin the Battle of the Bulge. When the going gets rough and you feel as if you will die without that piece of pecan pie, remember that no battle is ever easy or fought without sacrifice. The diary is your battle plan.

6 How Many Calories Do You Need Each Day?

or, Midriff Mathematics

One of the easiest methods of determining how many calories you need is to multiply the number of pounds you wish to weigh by a number from 11 to 15. If you want to weigh 175, and are moderately active—which means you get some form of exercise nearly every day—multiply 175 by 15. Your daily calorie allowance is then 2,625. Office workers or a homemaker should probably rate themselves a 12 or 13, and people who are not active at all, an 11. If you are a construction worker or otherwise expend enormous amounts of energy frequently, give yourself a 17. If you do not have a great deal of weight to lose, you could try cutting back your calories immediately to your approximate calorie allowance, but if you need to be a big loser, it is best to pick a midpoint, say what you might safely weigh in six months, and work from that. But do not set an unrealistic goal that you cannot meet, for failing to meet your goal will only drive you into depression—and probably the kitchen! Research indicates that the longer it takes you to lose weight, the longer the weight will stay off.

• Add up the calories you consume during a week-long period. Divide by seven. Now you have an approximate daily calorie intake; from that subtract what your intake, as figured above, should be. You'll see the number of calories you need to cut back in order to lose weight. Thus if your daily intake is 3,000, and you are a five-foot-five secretary, you are consuming nearly twice the amount of calories you should be for your optimum weight. We don't want this to seem like advanced mathematics, but if you are going to sustain a new eating pattern, you have to take responsibility for it yourself.

• If you find you are consuming the approximate number of calories that you have estimated to be right for you but are still overweight, you may have figured your activity rating too high, and should switch to a lower number. *Something* is causing the flab to stay put.

Determining your intake and burn-off of calories will show you how physical activity will help you stay slim. While it is true that exercise alone is not going to allow you to lose the amount of weight you wish (in all likelihood), it can and will make an enormous difference over a period of time. For each 3,500 calories you subtract from your life, you will lose a pound. Let's say you start to jog three times a week, until you are up to three miles each time. Since each mile covered uses up approximately 100 calories, you are burning off 900 calories a week that you weren't before—more than half a pound each week. That may not sound like much, but over twelve weeks that's six more pounds you wouldn't have lost. And we haven't even mentioned the additional benefits—improved muscle tone, a sense of well-being, cardiovascular improvement. A body works best when it's used. There's lots more on exercise, but this is just to give you an idea of how increased movement can make the numbers game easier.

7 The Attack on Overeating

or, The Menu Is Your Battle Plan

For the next two or three weeks, plan exactly what you are going to eat each day. Select the foods, total up the calories, and work out your own diet. Yes, this may require more thinking than simply going on someone else's diet, but you should begin to work out your own plan to accommodate your needs, your preferences. Remember you are working out a new plan for your life. . . . Why should you borrow someone else's?

However, if the thought of doing this alone right at the beginning seems overwhelming, find a diet that seems to suit your needs and stick to that for a time. Make sure it is well balanced (not overly high in protein or fats, no matter how popular the diet is) and one with which you feel comfortable. For some people, it is easiest to diet when they follow a battle plan to the letter, but what you are trying to do this time is work out a new diet for your life; and you aren't always going to have a half grapefruit and a slice of dry toast for breakfast, are you?

• Your diet should always include foods you find palatable, including ones that are your favorites; otherwise it won't work. You'll feel deprived and sorry for yourself, and be inclined to binge to get back at the diet and the quirk of fate that made you fat in the first place.

• As we will explain in Chapter 16, "Food and Nutrition," the American diet is overloaded with protein, and you will find it easier in the long run to slim down if your diet includes a goodly amount of complex carbohydrates. We don't mean cakes and pies but foods like beans, brown rice, whole grain breads, corn, potatoes, pasta—all those things you thought you shouldn't touch. Not only do they fill you up, they keep you feeling full for a long time. That's because they enter the bloodstream evenly over several hours, helping to prevent the problems many dieters experience—insomnia, irritability, lightheadedness, lack of energy, and, yes, that hungry feeling.

• Keep your calorie book next to you when you are planning the meals for the week. Look up every item. Take a calorie counter with you when you go shopping and check before you buy. Some items will have the caloric value on the package. Stay away as much as possible from canned goods. Head for the fresh vegetables. If you can't shop often or fresh vegetables are limited, buy frozen. Plain vegetables. You don't want those mixtures with sauces—that's where the sugar and fats are.

• Buy a new place setting: silverware, plates, place mat, glass, the works—and eat only with them. It will remind you that you are eating in a new way. You will be less tempted to "cheat" on these new dishes than the old ones on which you are used to overeating.

• You might select a thin person you know as your model eater. Note exactly what he or she does and imitate. Does he put his knife and fork down between each bite? Does he cut his pieces daintily? Does he take an animated part in the conversation? Does he thoroughly chew each bite? Now try it yourself. Again and again. When you are with company, with your family, and, yes, even alone.

8 Mind Games

or, Psych Up to Slim Down

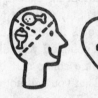 We're giving you plenty of rules and ideas on how you might go about changing your life to help you reach your goal of a new thin you. But you will only heed the advice if you want to. Can you help yourself want to? Can you make yourself want to so badly that you can walk by Baskin-Robbins without even a fleeting thought of a double mint chocolate chip cone? Certainly. There are specific mind games that will let you exercise your willpower over the old pattern of *mangia, mangia!*

• In your food diary, write down how you feel about being fat. When and how you got that way. When you put on extra pounds. How the people around you reacted to your gaining weight. Is the rest of your family fat? Were you a fat baby? Chubby in grade school? Why do you stay fat? Are you afraid of losing weight? In short, put down anything in your life that you can think of that relates to your weight. Just writing it down will help clarify your feelings and strengthen your resolve.

• On another page note the things you do that keep you fat.

We're not only talking about food. Write down ways in which you get out of exercising that could be changed.

• And on yet another page, put down a single number: what you want to weigh in a year. Say it to yourself when you feel a binge coming on.

• In the morning, set aside fifteen extra minutes before you get up. Lie quietly in a comfortable position and count to ten, all the while telling yourself to relax, relax. Do not move. Tell your body to relax while you keep your mind alert. When you are totally relaxed physically, imagine in your mind's eye a picture of the new thin you. What you will look like. What you will say. How you will act. What kind of clothes you will be wearing. Put yourself anywhere you want to be—at work, in the Caribbean, dancing at the hot new disco, meeting someone at a party. Stay with the picture. Tell yourself that this new thin you is yours for the asking; all you must do is get through the day without going off your diet. Tell yourself that you will not overeat. That the coffee cart bell with not signal a Danish and a cup of coffee. That you will not eat two bags of chips on the way home from work. That you will not have two drinks after work. Tell yourself that today will be a thin day, no matter what yesterday was like. Tell yourself that you deserve this chance at a new life because you are worth the trouble. In other words, talk to yourself about your diet, picture yourself as thin. You may wish to spend more than fifteen minutes with this exercise because it is so relaxing. When you feel that enough time has passed, start coming out of the reverie by counting backward from ten. When you reach *one,* tell yourself that when you awake you will be *wide awake* and you know what? You will be. And you won't feel like eating much.

• For a refresher during the day, try to steal even five minutes alone and in peace. If you have an office, close the door and take the phone off the hook. Sit back and do a short version of the above exercise. Then go to lunch.

• Dying, absolutely dying, for a piece of cheesecake from the bakery downtown that makes it divinely? Okay, have it, but *eat it in your mind*. Imagine getting in the car right now and driving downtown. How's the traffic? Did you make the light? Park the car. Get out and walk into the store. My goodness, doesn't it smell great? Look at all those cookies! Pastries! Sweet buns! Pies! And over there . . . is the cheesecake! Ask the girl for the whole thing. Watch her take it out of the display case and wrap it. Pay for it and leave. Drive home with it on the seat next to you. Bring it inside and cut yourself a nice big piece. Take it over to the table and sit down. Dig in. Taste the creamy smooth filling, the soft crust. Does it have a sour cream topping? Mmmm. Eat slowly, relishing every single crumb. Have another bite. And another. Have as many as you would like. Eat the whole pie if you like. Does this sound a little crazy? Perhaps. But somewhere along the line you will discover that you no longer crave cheesecake or whatever because you have already consumed it *in your mind*. There will even be times when as soon as you get the first bite into your mouth, you will feel satiated. This sounds odd, but trust us. Try it and see if it doesn't get you through some rough moments.

• Throughout the day—anyplace, anytime—stop for a second and think a thin thought about yourself. Think: How I will look next summer in a bathing suit. Think: Won't my boss be impressed when he sees that I've lost 50 pounds? Think: After I lose the weight, I'm going to ask Susie or Judy or Rita for a date. Think: After I lose the weight, I'm going to buy clothes from that boutique around the corner that doesn't carry a thing over size 12. Think: Someday I'm going to wear elegant Italian suits. Think: Anything you want. Doing this throughout the day will motivate you to stay with your new plan for eating, your new plan for your life.

9 Rewards

or, What Am I Going to Get Out of This?

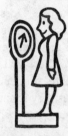 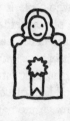 For starters, there's a new body. Along with the usual complement of renewed self-confidence, increased energy, and a whole new wardrobe, more than likely. It's not all that easy to alter pants from size 16 to 6, and who wants to anyway? The idea of white pants has never been more appealing than after you've just lost weight.

But you need money, right? Why not set up a system of systematic rewards for yourself. You know you deserve it. You might decide to give yourself a quarter or fifty cents each day you stay in control, a dollar or more for every single pound you lose. Or simply put aside the money you would spend on junk food. Put it in a bank and plan to use the money for something nice for yourself—an article of clothing, a new plant for your room, a bunch of daisies in the middle of February.

Buying yourself a case of Reese's Peanut Butter Cups is not such a good idea.

• This business of giving yourself a reward may seem like a nice extra that you needn't indulge in, but it can have a powerful effect on your rate of loss and how well you stick to your diet plan. Several studies have shown that positive reinforcement—a perk for doing something the right way—is a stronger conditioning technique to assure that you will do it again than punishment for doing something wrong. So pat yourself on the back for every single goal you reach while losing weight. You have probably spent years deriding yourself for being out of control and overweight.

• One woman we know had a willing mate who agreed to do a favor for her for every half pound she lost. He would give her a back rub, do the dishes, drive the kids to the skating rink on Saturday—anything within reason. And how nice to know you're loved.

• Stop anybody who tries to compliment you when you know you don't deserve it. Nothing can be so undermining as being complimented when there is nothing really to compliment you for. Stop the do-gooders in their tracks—say "thanks, but I haven't lost a pound since I saw you"—otherwise when you really have lost weight, you won't believe the praise.

• Do something nice for your body. A massage at the gym? A manicure? A new hairstyle? A cut at a salon you've always wanted to go to but thought was too expensive? There will never be a better time to reward yourself than now. Never.

• And what happens if you slip up for a day? *Absolutely nothing*. You are not going to be whipped at the post and so don't do it to yourself mentally either. If you are like most fat people, you have been down on yourself for years. More of that you don't need. Shrug and let it pass by. Tomorrow is another day, a new beginning.

10 Getting Rid of the Booby Traps in Your Home

or, Is There a Cookie Jar under Your Bed?

Most of our eating goes on in our own homes, so it makes sense not to have the place booby-trapped with food cues, ones that we have learned to respond to in the past. Time to clean house!

• Do you have a cookie jar filled with snacks so the kids can always have something to nibble on? Are you one of the "main" nibblers? Explain to your family what you are doing—and move the cookie jar out of sight. Put it in the cabinet. In a closet. Or better still, do away with it altogether! Fill it with noodles or dog bones.

• There are a zillion different things you can paste to your refrigerator door. Our suggestion: Use more than one and change them weekly. If you get used to seeing a picture of the fat you taped to the door, you will stop *really* seeing it. Your eyes will pass over it as just another part of the scenery. Here are a few ideas:

—A picture of you looking your worst
—A picture of you when you were thin
—A picture of someone famous you admire who is thin
—Slogans, such as "now really . . ."; "Are you hungry?"; "Don't forget to put it in your diary"; "Why not have it later?"; "Remember, last week at this time you weighed _____." You get the idea.
—A picture of a model wearing an outfit you especially like, something you wouldn't dream of wearing now
—A picture of something you are going to reward yourself with when you have lost a certain number of pounds. It's best to plan lots of rewards, and give them to yourself for every few—say five—pounds. That way the diet seems manageable.
—A mirror

• Do you snack every time you clean house in the afternoon? Do it in the morning. Do something else in the afternoon. Go for a walk, go window shopping, but get out of the house if you can.

• Do you snack when you pay your bills at the kitchen table? Pay your bills in another room. Stay out of the kitchen.

• Buy an article of clothing that you are looking forward to wearing, but one that is for your ideal weight, not the way you are now. Hang it outside the kitchen door so that you have to pass it every time you enter.

• Keep snack foods for other members of the family in a place where you don't have to see them every time you cook dinner. Out of sight long enough, and they will be out of mind.

• Repackage your food into smaller portions. Say that you decide that every now and then you are going to have a few cookies. Buy them, bring them home, and rewrap them into packages of two or three. That way you can have a package of cookies, but will be less tempted to have another. Those few seconds when you have to stop and think about what you are doing will help you resist. Think: Am I really hungry or am I just stuffing myself?

• Put leftovers in containers you can't see into. You'll feel less tempted to wolf down a few spoonsful of cold spaghetti if you don't see it every time you open the refrigerator door.

• Freeze leftovers and use them for another meal. Did you ever notice how after supper you would say to yourself—there's enough for lunch tomorrow—but by the time tomorrow got there, there wasn't? But you'll be less tempted to go to the trouble of defrosting something and heating it when it's just for a snack.

• Tell yourself again and again: There is nothing wrong with throwing food away. That little bit on your child's plate—too little to save, but I could just pop it into my mouth . . . really? And who is that going to help? The starving children in China?

• And if you give in to that almond-studded coffeecake when you are shopping, but after a few bites (at home—not in the car!) it doesn't seem worth all the calories and the way you feel about yourself—*throw it out!* If you keep it around and have only a small piece every day, you will still have consumed all the calories in it. If you throw out a coffeecake today, it's unlikely you'll go out and buy another one tomorrow.

• If you have leftovers from a party, can you seal them up and save them for another party? Peanuts can be stashed, Swedish meatballs can be frozen, stale chips can be thrown out. If you think of the food as being reserved for a special purpose, you will be less tempted to snack on it.

• Take an inventory of the food at home. Do you need all that? Do you keep food around for guests who might drop in? Are they foods you like? Do you keep cookies for the kids, for the neighbors, for your spouse? And nothing for poor little you? Admit you keep those foods around because you like them. And then use them up—or throw them out—and do not replace them.

• Bring less food into the house.

• Even though a teaspoon of sugar has only 18 calories, you will usually use much more than that on cereal or in coffee. If you must use sweetener, fill the sugar bowl with artificial sweetener, but always keep trying to cut down. It's the habit of always having to have everything taste sweet that you're trying to break—for a lifetime.

11 Hitting the Supermarket

or, Success at the Front Lines

Unless you decide that from now on you are going to have all your food delivered after you order it on the telephone, you are going to be faced with wheeling a shopping cart past rows and rows of goodies that you have not done without in ages. You know what your downfalls are, and you know exactly where they are stashed in your favorite supermarket. It will seem odd the first time you come home without herring in cream sauce or a sour cream poundcake or a quart of mint chocolate chip, but take heart—eventually it will be easy. Practice makes perfect. Or nearly so.

The most important thing about shopping is to prepare for it before you step through the door. Don't find yourself walking across the parking lot and thinking . . . now what should I get? You shouldn't be doing that anyway, since you are now planning your meals in advance. In addition to saving yourself calories, you save cash, since the items you are likely to buy on impulse are the high-ticket items.

• Prepare your shopping list when you plan your menus. Ideally, you'll work out what you will eat for a few days at a time in advance. That will let you have the freshest fruits and vegetables, which not only retain the greatest amounts of vitamins and minerals, but look the most appetizing. Food doesn't have to be boring on any diet; in fact, take special care to see that it does look appealing. You want to really enjoy what you eat, not wolf it down hardly aware of taste, color and texture.

• Plan your meals—and the shopping list—when you are not hungry. Just after a meal is the best time.

• Take your brand-name calorie book to the store with you. Comparison shop.

• Don't shop when you are hungry. You'll be feeling low, and when you pass those chocolate bars, you'll want one twice as badly as you would otherwise. Shop only when you are full, calm —and in charge of the situation! People who shop on a full stomach purchase between 10 and 20 percent less groceries than those who shop hungry.

• Shop first for produce. Load up on fresh fruit and vegetables.

• Buy all canned fruits packed in natural juice. Because the message that not all of America wants sugar in nearly everything is finally getting across to the food processors, some national brands are now packing certain items without added sugar. Pineapple and apple sauce are two such items now easy to find.

• *Do not eat in the supermarket.* No matter how tempting it seems. How would you feel if you ran into someone who knows about your new program?

• Buy tuna packed in water.

• When you buy pickles, make sure they don't contain any sugar. READ THE LABEL OF EVERYTHING THAT GOES INTO YOUR BASKET.

• Although butter and margarine have the same amount of calories, margarine is generally better for you since it contains no cholesterol, and polyunsaturated oils and margarines actually help you get rid of excess cholesterol—if you select carefully. What you want is the highest ratio of polyunsaturates to saturates. The label should list "liquid" vegetable oil and name the kind—safflower, soybean, or corn as the first ingredient. Best bets: tub margarine or those that come in a bottle or tube.

• And when you have decided to treat yourself, buy smaller packages of high-calorie foods, even though the cost per ounce is higher. You will probably end up spending less money in the long run. If you buy a bag of chips that you must have *just this once,* you will eat a lot more per sitting—if not demolish the whole bag— than if you purchase a smaller, more-expensive-per-ounce bag. Ditto with cookies, Fritos, chocolate bars.

• Look for low-sugar jellies and jams. They aren't all in specially marked diet containers.

• If you must buy commercially prepared salad dressings, choose the low-oil kind. Better: a mixture of yogurt or buttermilk and garlic, maybe some dill.

• Stick to oatmeal, Ralston, or Wheatena or plain shredded wheat when choosing a breakfast cereal. They have no added sugar or salt or chemicals you can't pronounce. Even those brands touted for their nutritional content have surprisingly high amounts of sugar. Read the label. Remember, ingredients are listed in order of their quantity.

• If you are going to bake a treat (for the children, naturally), buy the ingredients only when you know you are *actually going to bake.* Having all the ingredients on hand for chocolate chip cookies (walnuts, chocolate chips) is an open invitation to snack on them. No!

• Buy plain yogurt and add your own fresh fruit or low-calorie jams and jellies. A half teaspoon of vanilla and a bit of sweetener can turn plain yogurt into a yummy dessert.

• Buy skim milk mozzarella cheese. It's great for snacking.

• Look over the fresh fish before heading for the meat counter. Fish contains fewer calories than even chicken and veal, and should be a staple on every diet menu. It's loaded with vitamins and minerals and, except for a few varieties, is low in fat. Salmon, sardines, swordfish, and shad have more fat than most.

• Diet mayonnaise has less than half the calories of the regular kind—which has about a hundred per tablespoon.

• Be aware that not all "diet" foods have fewer calories than others. Some actually are higher in calories than the regular type. Most "diet" foods will save calories, of course, but make sure. For example, an 8-ounce can of Libby's beef stew contains 154 calories, while an 8-ounce can of Dia-Mel beef stew contains 200 calories. And a Stella D'Oro peach-apricot pastry contains 99 calories, while their dietetic peach-apricot pastry contains 104.

• Pass right by the "diet" soda. It's high in salt and contains as

〰〰〰〰〰〰〰〰〰〰〰〰〰〰〰〰〰〰〰〰〰〰〰〰〰〰〰

Coping with the Dieter's Blues

During the first week of any diet you are likely to feel weak, tired, perhaps even slightly nauseated. You might get a dull headache. This should pass by the second week. To ward off the blahs, make sure the diet has sufficient salt, lack of which can cause irritability and depression, and potassium, without which your muscles tend to cramp. High-potassium foods include: spinach, bananas, tomatoes, Brussels sprouts, flounder, and orange juice. If your particular diet has cut out all salt and you feel fatigued and low, try adding just a pinch of it. True, your weight loss might be slowed a bit, but you'll be more likely to stick to the diet.

〰〰〰〰〰〰〰〰〰〰〰〰〰〰〰〰〰〰〰〰〰〰〰〰〰〰〰

much phosphorus as the sugary kind—and excessive phosphorus drains calcium from your bones.

• Take a photograph of yourself everywhere with you—either a shot of the fat or the skinny you. When you find yourself reaching for those chocolate bars, stop and take a peek at it.

12 Partners in Crime or Friends?

or, How to Turn <u>Nearly</u> Everyone into a Thin Person's Ally

Sadly, there are people around who are going to try to sabotage your plan for a new you. Some of them won't mean to interfere—they're only doing what they are used to, like making that special strudel that you loved as a kid when you come to visit. But some of the people who will hinder your weight loss know, either consciously or unconsciously, exactly what they are doing.

Your spouse may worry that if you lose weight, you may leave. A husband may worry that if his wife suddenly becomes attractive, he'll have to deal with a whole new person. Say he takes her to the annual Christmas party. When she was fat, he never had to worry that any of the other men might flirt, but now what? And a wife may feel that her new, slim husband won't find her quite as attractive as he did before. It is best to deal with these problems head-on; instead of wondering why your spouse keeps bringing you

chocolate eclairs on the way home from work, confront him with
the issue and reassure him that your aim is to lose weight, not end
a marriage. With friends, lovers, and relatives who expect you to
go on acting like the old fat you, it's wise to take the bull by the
horns and get them—if you can—to work with, rather than against,
you. Remember, great wars were not won by one man (or
woman) alone.

• If your mate keeps bringing home fattening foods when he or
she didn't before, ask how your dieting affects him or her. Are
they annoyed because there is only diet food in the house? Have
you become irritable? Less interested in sex? Don't confront your
partner with hostility ("Why are you trying to sabotage me?"),
but deal with his or her feelings.

• When you are invited for lunch or dinner at a restaurant, say
in advance that you are on a diet and will be eating lightly, but
emphasize that you want to get together with the other person.
"I'll be ordering fish or a salad wherever we go, and so why don't
you pick the place?"

• Some of your toughest opponents are going to be the people
who know and love you best. When you reject their food, they are
going to feel that you are rejecting their love. A long, serious dis-
cussion about what you are doing will clear the air. Say you know
that you have been on diets before, and always gained the weight
back, but this is different. You are not simply going on a diet, you
are changing your life. Tell them you know it is going to be hard
on you, and you need the help and support of everyone. Ask them
not to suggest a piece of chocolate cream pie since you have been
doing so well lately on the diet. A compliment, a movie, a book
you have been wanting are the kinds of rewards you need now.

• Perhaps you will be able to diet with a friend. Someone who
doesn't think you are crazy when you call in the middle of a chocolate attack. Someone with whom you can place friendly bets.
You could bet $10 a week over who will lose more. Two people
we know each lost between $150 to $170, but each won nearly all

of the money back. The $10 just kept going from one to the other. One study found that a friend is actually a better dieting companion than a mate, for the mate is likely to have an emotional investment in your staying the same, while a friend is not. Those who dieted with a friend actually lost nearly twice as much as those who enlisted the help of a spouse.

● If you can't find a dieting partner—and only a lucky few will—ask someone to be your ally through the hard part of the diet. Someone with whom you can share your hopes, aims, and aspirations. Someone you can trust. He or she can be there to cheer you on with your successes or be supportive when the going gets rough. Sharing your frustrations and fears can put them into their proper perspective and make them seem less ominous. Sometimes just talking them out will make them evaporate.

● Ask your ally to offer suggestions along the way, such as "Do you really need two sugars in your coffee?"; "Why don't you try the green beans with just lemon juice instead of butter?"; and "You don't really want potato chips, do you?" The friend shouldn't be your warden, but someone who will deliver the message in a warm and loving way.

● Pick an ally who is thin. You can hardly expect someone who's 50 pounds overweight and not ready to go on a diet to be very sympathetic to your efforts. It will make that person seem out of control and resent you for even asking.

● Be prepared to hear comments like "You've lost too much weight—you look tired all the time!" and "I don't know how to deal with you anymore—you're always counting calories. We can't even enjoy a meal out anymore!" And the killer: "I liked you better when you were fat." Try not to be nasty and try to be patient with these people. Eventually, they will come to appreciate the new thin you. But maybe not everybody will. Remember that you cannot be all things to all people, and that there will always be people who do not like you, whether it's the fat you or the thin you.

• A lot of people play a game with dieters. It's called "How Do I Make X Go Off the Diet?" You will be asked once if you want something to eat. No, you say. You will be asked again. And again. No, you repeat, trying to be as diplomatic as you can. Say things like "I know your cake (candy, sauce, whatever) looks absolutely divine, and I'm sure it tastes the same way. But I'm on this new program, you see, and I know if I take just a little I will want a lot more, so I'd just as soon have none today, but thanks anyway." That may still not quiet your adversary. But if you give in, you will resent the other person. You probably won't explode over a single spongecake or slice of pizza, but you may store up the resentment for future use, and when the other person again offers something you don't want to eat, you may explode like Mount Saint Helens. Warn your friends ahead of time. That should stop the proffering of puff pastry. And remember that it is always best to assert yourself as events occur, deal with your anger as it comes up. Any kind of emotion is easier to handle in small doses.

• Say you know you are going to have dinner at your Aunt Clara's. She is absolutely famous for her cheesecake. After dinner, which hasn't been a bender as far as calories are concerned, you are quite sure she's going to spring one of her cheesecakes on you. You have always eaten them with gusto, to say the least, having not just one but two or three pieces. You can visualize the scene. You can also plan in advance how you will deal with the situation. Be tactful, try not to hurt her feelings, but get your point across.

When she says that you've been on diets before and they never worked, tell her this is different.

When she says that you always loved her cheesecake—ever since you were a little kid and now what's wrong, tell her that you love it more than ever, but you're an adult now and are going to have to pass on it today since you really want to lose weight this time.

When she says that she's noticed that you already look tired and drawn, tell her that's only because she's used to seeing your face filled out with fat.

Tell her you don't come to visit because she makes the best cheesecake, you come to see her because you like her.

When she asks what she's going to do with all that leftover cheesecake, suggest she freeze it for later or give it to her friends or the kids next door.

After your dinner with Aunt Clara, and resisting the cheesecake, you will feel as if you deserve a medal. And you do! Changing your behavior is always difficult for those around you to understand—until they get used to it.

• Dealing with your parents may prove to be the stickiest situation yet, because no matter how old you are, you are still the child. And that's how they are going to treat you. Ever wonder why you eat and eat and eat when you go to visit? It's because they spent all those years feeding you, and during the process love and food became forever entwined. No matter what they think of you today, you want to please them, just like a child, by licking your plate clean. Your mother bakes for weeks ahead of your annual visit—how can you turn down the food?

Ask yourself: Must I still act like a child? Must my parents dictate how much I eat? Explain the situation to your family, but be aware you will still have to stick to your guns. Many a mother mistakenly equates your love for her with how much you can shovel in.

• If you see your parents frequently, turn some of the situations around: Invite them over to your place. There you can dictate what's put on the table. What to do with the food your mother brings may still pose a problem, but not as much as when you see her toiling over that hot kitchen stove. Remember, you can always give it away. The kids on the block or the elderly lady who lives alone will probably be thrilled with a surprise strudel.

• Take your parents to a restaurant. Not only will you be able to select the place, one where you know you can eat without drowning yourself in creamy sauces, they may be pleased with the idea of such an outing with their son or daughter as the host. It's the kind of thing that's nice to tell the neighbors about. "Our son Jim took us out for the nicest dinner last night. . . ."

• If you are at home for an extended stay, try eating a few meals elsewhere. Go out and visit a friend when lunch might be served; stay in bed late and make a light breakfast for yourself. Since skipping meals entirely is not a good idea, don't use it as a last-ditch solution to the parent problem. Instead you might go for a walk during lunch and take along a piece of fruit, a small wedge of cheese.

• Then there's dinner at some friends' house. Depending on the relationship, you have two choices. Call the hostess or host in advance and explain the situation. Say you will be eating less than usual, and would appreciate not being asked to have seconds. Say you know they are good cooks, but you don't want to gorge yourself and hate yourself and them the next morning when you step on the scale. That works if you know the people quite well.

If you don't (dinner at the boss's house would not be such a place to use the above ploy), there is nothing to do but go to the meal and *eat lightly*. They won't know that you usually take three helpings of mashed potatoes anyway, and aren't likely to force food on you. Resolve beforehand that you will limit yourself to a certain number of drinks—say one. Period. That you will put everything on your plate and take a polite bite or two of the fattening foods and push the rest around to make it look as if you are eating it. Concentrate on eating whatever has the fewest calories. If you can get away with forgoing the dessert, do so. If not, dawdle over your food. No one is going to tell you about the starving millions in India, or say that you are a naughty child because you didn't clean your plate.

• Remember to be enthusiastic in your praise of the baked Alaska or whatever. "I'm so full that I can't eat another bite, but this is delicious!" Then change the subject.

• In all situations when you have to eat outside the home, take a moment and rehearse in your mind how you will act. Practice saying, "No thanks, I couldn't eat another bite." You needn't stop your life—you can do this while getting ready and while driving there. Running through the scene ahead of time gives you practice on how to act with your new behavior. You might also want to think over how your hosts might respond, and practice refusing any pressure.

• Promise yourself that before going to bed after a dinner party or a meal with your parents, you will step on the scale. Sure, you know that you weigh more after a meal, but the question is: how much more?

• Tell yourself just before you step out the door that you too can be assertive. Fat people with a low self-image have a hard time standing up for themselves. When someone says "Eat!" tell yourself you don't have to—be militant—then (less militantly), tell them.

• And now—enjoy yourself. You'll probably find that the dinner conversation is more stimulating than you remember. That's because before you were too busy to take an active part in the table talk.

13 How to Eat Like a Thin Person

or, Table Techniques

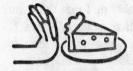

- Drink a glass of water before each meal. Or have an apple ten minutes before dinner. You will feel full and won't overeat.

- Sit at the table for a full minute before you start eating. It will help you practice willpower.

- Cut the food into small pieces. Even a banana.

- Chew each mouthful ten times.

- Put down your knife and fork between bites. Really taste the food.

- TALK, TALK, TALK. You can't talk with a full mouth. It slows down the consumption, gives your stomach time to inform the brain that you are getting full.

- Select foods that take longer to eat; you'll pile away less. Eat a baked potato rather than mashed, for example, and eat less of it; eat raw fruit rather than custard. Have a big green salad—fewer calories to start with—instead of easy-to-scoop-up macaroni and cheese.

• Don't save the best for the last. You will want to eat it anyway. Have you ever noticed how you "couldn't eat another thing—except dessert"?

• Eat the food highest in nutrition first. Your stomach is best able to digest what it gets first.

• If possible, always sit down at a buffet dinner. You'll eat more standing up without realizing when you have put away enough calories. If you eat standing up you may fool yourself into thinking you haven't eaten much of anything.

• Try eating with the opposite hand.

• When you've had it with carrot sticks and zucchini strips, try the "taste" method. It works like this: You order broiled fish and fresh fruit at a restaurant, but "taste" your companion's salmon mousse and peach melba. One bite only!

• Do not eat anything that is boring. If you don't like what you are eating, you won't feel satisfied and you'll want to gorge later.

• A tablespoon of gravy goes further if you put it next to—not on—your meat. Dip a corner of your piece into the sauce.

• If you are going to indulge with Roquefort, don't waste it on wilted lettuce. Save it for the best.

• Eat vegetarian. Start with once a week. If you take time and care to prepare attractive and nutritious meals, you'll probably soon be doing it two or three times a week. You'll almost always consume fewer calories, less fat.

• Try rabbit. The meat is all white, high in protein, and contains less fat and fewer calories per ready-to-cook pound than chicken, veal, beef, or pork. The French eat it regularly. The French are not known for fatness either.

• Never let yourself get too hungry between meals. If a meal is delayed past four hours or so from the last one, have a snack—

plain yogurt, a little water-packed tuna, a slice of turkey breast, a piece of fruit.

• Serve yourself several courses to make your meal seem like more and give your brain time to get the message that you are full. Have a cup of broth, the main course, a salad, then fruit.

• Pile up your salad plate. High. Sprinkle with lemon juice.

• Second helpings are for growing kids, not you.

• Slow down!

14 Eating Alone

or, Staying in Control Even Though No One's Watching

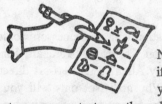

Nearly every single behavior-modification program recommends that you do nothing else while you eat. That you concentrate on the colors and textures and tastes of the food you are eating. That you dine. That you pay attention to when you feel full—how are you even going to know when hunger is satisfied if you are watching "The Waltons"?

If you have been eating without paying attention, it's easy to understand why you have become a compulsive calorie consumer. It will be necessary to backtrack and turn each meal into a dining event.

But we know some of you won't give up dining with the evening news or your book. If you live alone, eating as pure experience—nothing else going on at the same time—may seem terribly restrictive and actually punishing. So you are on your own on this one. You may decide that you need—at least for a time—to do nothing during meals except *eat,* and if so, go right ahead. You're on the side of the behavior-modification people who practically have this rule written in blood. But if you decide to take the other course—not give up reading or watching television while you eat—arm yourself in other ways.

- Fix a nice dinner.

- Set a place for yourself at the coffee table if that's where you insist upon eating.

- Eat slowly and concentrate not only on what you are reading or watching, but what is going into your mouth.

- Don't automatically go back to the kitchen for more without asking yourself if you really want more.

- In the same way you would pause for conversational breaks if you were dining with someone, pause for reflection. Think about what you are seeing or hearing or reading. Put down your knife and fork for a minute.

- Have an imaginary conversation with someone you would like to meet, living or dead. Winston Churchill? Abraham Lincoln? Edna St. Vincent Millay? Woody Allen? That new art director at work you think is attractive? Why not? Not only will you keep your mind busy, but it will provide you with the opportunity to practice your conversational skills and even help you overcome your shyness later on.

You can beat the system. You can make your own.

15 Danger in the Kitchen

or, Snares in the Salads

 It's not your friendly neighborhood burglar we're talking about —it's you. It's where the kids' cookies are stored, where you prepare the meals, have a cup of coffee with the morning newspaper. But is it also where you pay your bills, watch television, and talk on the telephone? Going into the kitchen—for whatever reason—may provide you with a food cue. You're used to eating when you pass through, and so every time you step inside, your unconscious is telling you something like "Wouldn't a cookie taste good right now?" or "Maybe I'll just taste that leftover beef stew."

Now if you work at resisting the temptation long enough, the kitchen will no longer trigger an "I want to eat something" response the minute you pass through its portal. But until you get there, it's best to stay out as much as possible.

• Do correspondence in another room. If there's a phone in another room—always answer that one. Especially if it's upstairs. You'll get more exercise. Let the dog out another door. Put the TV in another room. Move the desk. And the sewing machine.

• If you're in charge of meals for a family, consider having them pitch in and help. There's no reason why you should have to chain yourself to the kitchen just because you have in the past. Maybe unconsciously you like to spend all that time cooking by yourself *because no one could catch you eating.* The burglar in the kitchen could be you, stealing your own good health and good looks.

• Ask your children to make their own lunches and snacks. If you explain why—that you are trying to learn a new behavior and until you've got it down cold, you need their help, they are likely to willingly help you reach your goal. They won't think that this means you don't like them enough anymore. Perhaps they can help you make dinner, too. A salad's not all that hard to handle. The more that others do with food, the less you'll have to.

• Ask somebody to keep you company while you're cooking. It takes calories to talk. And will you really feel like polishing off that piece of cold chicken in front of your child—whom you're always telling not to snack just before dinner because he'll ruin his appetite?

~~~~~~

Scaling the Plateau

If you lose weight the first week and don't the second—no matter how well you stick to your diet—don't despair. You have not been singled out to be fat forever. Most of the weight loss during the first week was water loss. During the second week, the body is struggling to regain equilibrium and is holding back on the water. Naturally, the standstill on the scale is frustrating, but remember: it will pass.

~~~~~~

To Taste or Not to Taste

• It's a rule of thumb that most good cooks taste their food as they prepare it. You can decide to do one of two things. Keep on tasting, but remember that you will have to add the calories in your daily total. Some people do so much "tasting" that they consume a few hundred calories before they get the meal on the table. A sip will do. And it need not be done over and over again. If you keep that up, you are only fooling yourself. And remember—just a hundred extra calories each day will put on 10 extra pounds during the course of a year.

• Or you can not taste at all. Most recipes are made with precise directions, and you can be quite sure that the food will taste as good as it's supposed to. And you know, the world won't end if the soup's not salted to everyone's taste. Others can add it at the table, and you will be doing everybody a favor by cutting back on salt.

• To keep you from munching while you're mincing, chew gum. Sugarless. Keep the pack visible to remind yourself. And before you start preparing any meal, remind yourself that thin people don't chow down while they cook, and you are on your way to becoming a thin person.

• If you must cook two separate dinners because people eat at different times, *do not eat both times*. This sounds so obvious that it may seem silly to mention it, but a lot of fatties feel it is their duty to eat with both groups of people so the others won't have to eat alone. *Fat people are always doing more for other people than themselves*. Take charge of your life, your time—and what you put into your mouth. No one will really be offended if you refuse to eat because you are going to eat later. On occasions when you feel this won't work—like the holidays with two sets of in-laws—eat twice if you must, but eat lightly. If you prepare an early meal for your children, and another for your husband and you, you shouldn't be called upon to eat with your children. Your children will find you just as good company if you sit and talk with them

~~~~~~

Did You Know . . .

that a porterhouse steak is more fat than protein by weight?

that the amount of water required to metabolize proteins is *seven times* greater than the amount needed by carbohydrates?

that a diet too high in proteins and fats will result in excessive water loss, which flushes out needed nitrogen, potassium, phosphorus, sulfur, and sodium?

that a medium-sized baked potato is about ninety calories and is a treasure-trove of vitamins, minerals, protein, and complex carbohydrates?

that the average American diet contains twice the amount of salt we need? And that it is a major contributor to high blood pressure? And that salt causes water retention?

that exercise decreases the amount of protein needed for good health?

that hard cheeses contain more saturated fat than beef?

~~~~~~

without a plate in front of you. Have your dinner with your spouse. A meal is a special time for the two of you. It's a time for conversation, for sharing the events of the day, and for sharing food. It is not a time for seeing how much you can stuff down.

• You may not realize you are eating two meals. You may think it's just a bite of this and a bite of that. But once you write it down in your food diary, you may learn that something quite different is occurring.

Remember, you are learning how to take control of your life. You are learning how not to let the situation get the best of you. You are learning how to be a thin person.

16 Food and Nutrition

or, You Mean I Really Can Eat Potatoes?

The Case for the Carbohydrate

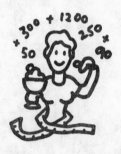

Contrary to popular belief, the best way to lose weight is not to go on a high-protein–low-carbohydrate regimen. You will lose more weight, feel better, and take off more fat tissue if your diet includes a high percentage of *complex carbohydrates*. Not only that, your body's internal workings will shift from that of a fat person to that of a slim person, which means that it will be easier to keep weight off once you have lost it.

Sound like the exact opposite of every diet you've seen in the last decade or so? It is. But many proponents of the healthy life have long advocated that we eat more complex carbohydrates: They keep the blood sugar level on an even keel (and a sinking blood sugar level makes you feel hungry), are easy on the liver, high in vitamins, and aid elimination. Besides, aren't there times when a cup of bean soup would be tremendously satisfying? Bean soup sticks to the ribs, after all.

And now researchers at the University of Virginia have proven what a lot of us have instinctively known all along, even if the trendy diets kept us from acting on it: The body does best on a high-carbohydrate regimen. Now, admittedly, their work was done with rats—and not people—but the evidence is striking.

Two groups of rats were fed approximately the same number of calories each day. One group had 25 percent of its calories in protein, and the other group only had 5 percent protein. Both groups had approximately 10 percent of their calories in fat. The difference was made up in carbohydrates.

At the end of eight weeks, the high-protein group weighed *over 20 percent more* than the low-protein group! The body weight of the high-protein group was comprised of nearly 24 percent fat, while the other group had only 15 percent of its weight accounted for in fat tissue.

The researchers speculated that the low-protein diet may have produced more body heat, resulting in a natural burning off of calories, or that high protein diets deposit more calories in fat tissue than carbohydrates do.

Athletes who need endurance have long known that eating complex carbohydrates—not meat—for three days before the big race will give them that extra bit of energy near the finish line. And if it can help athletes, why not us, even if we're not running in a marathon?

The reason a diet high in carbohydrates helps you lose weight without that hungry feeling has to do with why you get hungry in the first place. When your blood sugar level (the amount of glu-

wwwwwwwwwwwwwwwwwwwwwwwwwwwwwwwwwwwwwwwwww

Sugar Fix

The average American consumes 126 pounds of sugar a year, most of it hidden in canned or processed foods. Mayonnaise, ketchup, frozen dinners, canned vegetables, and even cereals like cornflakes are laced with goodly amounts of that particular combination of carbon, oxygen, and hydrogen we call *sugar*.

wwwwwwwwwwwwwwwwwwwwwwwwwwwwwwwwwwwwwwwwww

~~~~~~

The Basics

* *Proteins* are found in: meats, poultry, fish, eggs, milk, cheese, nuts, seeds, beans, and grains.
* *Carbohydrates* are supplied by: fruits, vegetables, bread, cereals, grains, and sugars.
* *Fats* are plentiful in: whole-milk dairy products, fatty meats, egg yolks, nuts, and oils.

~~~~~~

cose circulating in your bloodstream) falls below a certain point, it triggers a mechanism in the brain that is transmitted to you as hunger.

However, when the blood sugar level exceeds a certain point—which can happen after a large meal or a sugary snack—insulin is released to lower the level by speeding the conversion of blood sugar to fat.

Eventually, your blood chemistry gets involved in a "fat" cycle. You eat sugar to get an energy *high;* but twenty minutes later, a *low* comes creeping in as an overdose of insulin floods the bloodstream and lowers the blood sugar. What happens? You feel hungry, naturally, and you reach for another shot of sugar.

But if you start eating in such a way to control that bouncing-ball syndrome, not only will you not have hunger pangs, your body will convert from having a fat person's metabolism to a thin person's, all of which will help you keep slim.

Chemically, a carbohydrate is any food containing carbon, hydrogen, and oxygen compounds. That includes all sugars, grains, legumes and other vegetables, fruits, and nuts. Meat, cheese, and eggs are mostly protein and/or fat; milk falls somewhere in between, since it contains carbohydrates as lactose or milk sugar, as well as protein and fat.

Now the kind of carbohydrates that are the best for us are the complex variety found in starches, legumes, vegetables, and milk. What the *complex* means is that the carbohydrate is mixed with a certain amount of protein or fat or both, and for the body to convert the carbohydrate into *glucose,* which is what the body uses for fuel, it must be separated from these other elements during digestion, all of which takes some time to occur. Glucose is released slowly and over a longer period of time into the blood-stream.

Complex carbohydrates, which are available aplenty in foods like starchy vegetables, whole-grain bread, cereals that haven't been refined to the point of no return, brown rice, beans of any sort, whole-wheat pasta, and bulgur wheat are the kinds of carbohydrates that are good for you, that keep the blood sugar level at an even keel. That's why that cup of lentil soup, which hasn't been on anybody's hit diet in years, is so satisfying. For 250 calories or so, it truly fills you up and keeps you from feeling hungry for a long time. Besides, the texture just feels comforting. The same is true of cooked or whole-grain cereals in the morning. If you haven't tried them for years, you will be surprised at how long you feel full.

Simple carbohydrates are those foods that are all carbohydrate, such as sugar (white, brown, raw, honey, molasses) and fruits; the carbohydrate in them is rapidly released into the bloodstream, causing a rapid rise in blood sugar, followed by a drop just as quickly. And you're hungry!

While fruit is a simple carbohydrate, the natural sweetness does not have the same effect on glucose levels as does sugar extracted from other foods. In addition, fruit provides fiber, vitamins, and minerals. But the amount of carbohydrate (10 to 15 grams per average piece) is nearly as bad as what you get in a single candy bar —up to 100 grams! Many nutritionists recommend that fruit be limited to one or two pieces a day, especially if you are hypoglycemic.

To further the case for carbohydrates, remember:

• They aid the liver in producing an adequate supply of glycogen, the substance that accounts for the blood sugar level, and adequate stores of glycogen in the liver make the body more resistant to insult from alcohol, arsenic, and bacterial toxins. Ever wonder why you crave things like pasta, cream soups, or tomato juice the morning after? It's your body trying to replenish carbohydrates.

• The liver is spared the job of taking apart amino acids and fatty acids, as it must when it gets glycogen from protein or fat. The liver doesn't really like to do this, and extra wear and tear on it are avoided *when the body has an adequate supply of carbohydrates.*

• A diet high in protein and low in carbohydrates causes the kidney to excrete toxic substances called ketones. If they build up in the blood, the individual may feel lightheaded, drowsy, cranky, apathetic, and nauseated and start to black out when rising quickly. Is this any way to feel when you're trying to adopt a new behavior pattern? Not on your life!

• And last but not least, a generous supply of carbohydrates reduces the dietary requirements for protein and what we are recommending is *not* expensive.

• The average American diet is 16.1 percent protein, more than twice the amount recommended for good nutritional health. Most of the protein we consume comes from meat and meat products, right? And that protein is often attached to fat. If you still need to be convinced that you probably eat too much protein, consider this: Researchers now know that high-fat diets and too much body fat *period* are related to an increased incidence of cancer.

• How many carbohydrates should you have daily? Somewhere between 100 and 110 grams spread throughout the day will keep blood sugar from dipping and give you more energy than usual. You won't experience the fatigue that is usually associated with losing weight, and many experts claim you will be better able to handle stress. And wouldn't that be nice, whether you're dieting or not?

● A study with obese young men on 1,800-calorie daily rations but with a varying amount of carbohydrates—104, 60, or 30 —found that the men who had 104 grams of carbohydrates lost more weight and fat tissue than the other groups. In addition, there was less loss of ketone bodies; hence, no blah feelings dieters often experience.

● Every now and then, you are probably going to have to allow yourself some favorite "treat"—damn the calories, damn the sugar! The idea that your life will not include one single more Hershey bar may just be too much for you. But remind yourself of this: If as little as 5 percent of your diet is in sugar calories, most likely you will still have a "sweet tooth" and will nearly always feel hungry. You've sent your blood sugar a reason to go skyrocketing—and then to plummet—and the message your brain will send is: MORE, MORE, MORE.

● What about when you're playing tennis, your energy is sagging, and you're behind? Should you take time out for a candy break? You need energy, after all. But by the time the candy is digested, the sugar sent to the liver, where the liver fusses with it and sends it out to the muscles, the game will have been won or lost. And you'll want another candy bar. Have an apple or a banana an hour before the game.

Fats

Fats are not totally bad guys, naturally. We have to have some in our diets. They help the body absorb certain vitamins (A, D, and E), keep our cells healthy, and form the protective sheath around nerves. They're necessary for a healthy skin and for the proper functioning of our reproductive organs. But nearly everybody today eats too much fat, and even if you were to cut out all the fat you imagine you are eating—give up bacon, hamburger, butter, cream, and so forth—you would still get plenty of fat in your diet. Cereals, fruit, and vegetables all contain a little fat.

Saturated and polyunsaturated fats—what do these terms mean? Fats are made up of three different types of acids—saturated, monounsaturated, and polyunsaturated, determined by how many places the molecule has available for extra hydrogen atoms. None? Saturated. Room for two? Monounsaturated. Can it take as many as four? Polyunsaturated.

Animal fats are mostly saturated fats. And all animal fat contains cholesterol. Coconut and palm oil—solid at room temperature—are higher in saturated fat than animal fat.

Peanut and olive oil are high in monounsaturates, and the vegetable oils that are high in polyunsaturates are cottonseed, soybean, and corn; sunflower and safflower are the highest in polyunsaturates. Sesame oil is split between polyunsaturates and monounsaturates.

The "prudent" diet recommended by many health organizations suggests that we try to consume more polyunsaturates than we currently do. Polyunsaturates and monounsaturates are perfectly capable of transporting fat-soluble vitamins, which is one of the major jobs of fat in our bodies. And all vegetable oils lack cholesterol.

Polyunsaturates tend to help the body get rid of unwanted cholesterol, and that's why they are the preferred choice. Peanut and olive oil don't make things worse, but they don't help either.

• The foods with the highest fat content will come as no surprise. Use these only sparingly: butter, lard, margarine, cooking oils, shortening, mayonnaise, fatty meats. Bacon and sausage are the worst offenders. Others are dairy products (except those marked low fat), duck, goose, avocado, olives, potato chips, and yes—chocolate. Unless you radically change your diet, you will continue to eat some of these items. The point is to start cutting back however you can.

• Switch to low-fat or nonfat milk. Just keep telling yourself it's good for your heart, it's good for your body, it will help keep you slim. Naturally, this doesn't give you license to drink a quart at each meal—or even a quart a day.

• Nuts are high in fat. If you feel you must have some, buy them in the shell. You'll probably consume fewer because it takes a little work to get to the kernel.

• Eggs have a lot of good things going for them—7 grams of protein—but are high in fat and cholesterol (250 milligrams per yolk). Limit yourself to no more than four a week. Some diets do away with them altogether.

• Avoid all processed meats like bologna, salami, and frankfurters. They're not only high in fat, they contain a number of chemicals that have no business in your body. If you like to buy sliced meats for sandwiches, try roasted turkey breast. It's available at a number of deli counters. Scores high in nutrition and low in fat. Did you know that turkey meat is good for the skin?

• Not only should you reduce the amount of fat overall in your diet, but also you should not overload at a single meal because you've deprived yourself for a week. Your liver will have a hard time processing all that fat at once.

Protein: Not the Dieter's Panacea

Notice we've turned the usual order of foods around? Put protein last? That's because we hear the most about it in this country (a tribute to the meat and dairy industries) and most of us have been brainwashed into believing we need gobs of it. Hogwash!

We all need some protein in our daily fare, but just how much is debatable and highly individual. While some people might do best on a high-protein diet, it is generally known that we need far less than we get—or is even recommended by the National Academy of Sciences.

The cells use protein to build various kinds of human protein: muscle, skin, hair, and blood. Without protein, new tissue needed for growth and replacement cannot be manufactured in the body; protein stimulates the production of antibodies and helps regulate the body's water and acid-base balance.

If it's so good, you ask, why are we knocking it? It's the way we are accustomed to thinking of protein today: red meat. Then fish and chicken. It is true that these animal proteins are "complete," in the sense that they contain all eight or nine of the essential amino acids the body requires, but the amount we consume, on the average, far surpasses our need. We all too often overlook grains, nuts, and vegetables as sources of protein. Eaten in the right combination, we can get adequate stores of protein from these sources—and we don't load down our bodies with the fat "baggage" that is a component of all animal protein.

The body would much rather use carbohydrates for energy, but when we choke it with too much protein and too few carbohydrates, it is forced to work harder to get the energy it needs from protein. Too much protein increases the need for fluids; that's why those high-protein diets suggest that you be sure to drink eight glasses of water a day to flush out the liver. In addition, excess protein speeds up the turnover of proteins in the body. This means the more you eat, the more quickly you need to replenish protein; the chain reaction speeds up the metabolic rate of the body, can shorten the life span of some cells, and may cause aging. Think of the body as a machine on "idle." Too much protein turns up the "idle" too high, just as when your automobile is set too high. You waste a lot of fuel. At the same time, the concentration of urea in the blood increases; in individuals with kidney or liver malfunction, urea can accumulate to such degrees that it can cause disorientation, coma, and even death. Which brings us back to the increased need for water when too much protein is consumed. Need more evidence that too much animal protein is bad—not good?

• Some sports doctors believe that every year a certain number of deaths occur during football practice due to dehydration. Young men trying to build themselves up on protein lose water, which prevents them from dissipating body heat, and they get heatstroke.

• Animal proteins produce higher cholesterol levels than vegetable proteins. When soybean, which nearly approximates animal protein in its balance of amino acids, was made a major component of a diet fed individuals with known high cholesterol levels, their cholesterol levels fell more than 30 percent, on the average.

One study found that even on a diet high in fat, serum lipids (fats) in the blood are reduced in persons consuming a large amount of vegetable protein.

• A recent study at the University of Wisconsin reports that diets high in protein significantly affect the calcium balance in the body. An individual who sharply increases his protein intake may find that what was once a sufficient amount of calcium in his diet is now inadequate to meet his needs. Sometimes the calcium needs are so high that the balance cannot be met.

This is especially crucial for women past thirty, for whom deficient calcium over a long period of time leads to a softening of the bones (osteoporosis). This can cause frequent breaks due to the bones' brittleness and fragility.

~~~~~~

Meaty Facts

Over the course of the twentieth century, complex-carbohydrate consumption has declined while that of refined starches and sugars has increased greatly. Fat consumption has actually dropped a bit and while our intake of protein has remained much as it was in, say, 1910, vegetables were then the main protein source, a place now assumed by meat. In the last three decades alone, our annual consumption of beef has risen from *55 pounds per person to 166 pounds,* and our consumption of poultry has gone from 16 pounds to 50! And yet we automatically groan every time we hear beef prices are rising. It may be a blessing in disguise, for Americans will start consuming less beef and look for alternate sources of protein. We hope. We hope you will.

~~~~~~

• At present, most Americans derive between 60 and 80 percent of their protein from animal sources. It is recommended that everyone—not just those on reducing diets—lower that amount to 35 percent and make up the deficiency from other sources. Pregnant women are an exception to the rule. But in general, adults need approximately the same amount of protein at age twenty as they did at age eight, and their needs decline steadily thereafter.

• The amount of protein your body requires is determined largely by age and weight. The National Academy of Sciences–National Research Council recommends a dietary allowance (RDA) of .8 gram of protein per kilogram of body weight per day for adults—46 grams for the average female, 56 grams for the average male. But wait: *This allows us nearly a third more than we actually need.* A safety factor was figured in; however, our feeling is that the percentage was far too generous. The United Nations Food and Agricultural Organization was more realistic and, considering what we need and what's available on a global scale, calculated with less abandon. Its protein recommendation: about a third less—and that is what is recommended by some nutritionists for optimum health—30 to 50 grams a day.

• For children, particularly infants who are extremely vulnerable to any imbalance in their diets, overabundant protein can be especially hazardous. Cow's milk—the basis of most formulas—contains twice the protein of human milk. It is not unusual for bottle-fed infants to be overfed and to start solid food early, and it is thought by some that many such infants may approach hypernatremic dehydration, a condition caused by water lost in flushing out a large waste load. This kind of dehydration is four times more deadly than the water loss that accompanies diarrhea in infants, and can lead to brain damage, kidney failure, and even death within hours.

• The Federal Trade Commission has come down hard on the promotion of protein for infants, because the average American infant consumes 18 percent of its calories as protein calories, and when that approaches 20 percent, the risk of dehydration is *1 to 2 percent*.

• High-protein diets for infants are thought to cause retention of urea, overtax the baby's immature kidneys, elevate the blood ammonia level, and cause the blood and other body fluids to be acidic.

~~~~~~

The Basic Food Groups

* Grains—breads, cereals, rice, and pasta
* Dairy products—milk, cheese, yogurt, butter
* Fruits and vegetables—including legumes, or beans
* Protein of animal origin—meat, fish, fowl, and eggs

~~~~~~

Select foods from each of the groups every day and you will have a variety of vitamins and minerals, carbohydrates, protein and fats, tastes, colors, and textures.

But you must also choose a variety of foods within each group. A friend of ours decided six months ago that broccoli was not only good, it was good for you, and now it's the vegetable he has with practically every single dinner he cooks. Last year it was spinach and succotash. All of them are good for you, but he would be doing better nutritionally if he switched around during the week—not just every year!

Protein Meals—Mostly Meatless

Since a single carbohydrate food will have some of the essential amino acids and lack others, the way to assure that you get all you need so your body can produce protein on its own is to eat carbohydrates in *combination*. What one lacks the other makes up. Here are some protein teams that work together:

Protein from Plants—Legumes and Grains

baked beans and brown bread
black-eyed peas and rice
beans and tortillas or cornbread
bean and barley soup
lentils and rice
lima beans and corn (succotash)
beans and noodles
peanut butter sandwich with whole-grain bread
refried beans and rice
chick peas and whole-grain bread
soybeans and noodles

Legumes with Seeds

green beans and almonds
peanuts and mixed nuts

One way to stretch the protein in your diet is to have a little of a meat or dairy product mixed with carbohydrates. The amino acids in the animal protein put a "spark" into the carbohydrates.

Protein from Animals and Grains

milk and cereal
cheese on pizza
cheese sandwich with whole-grain bread
macaroni and cheese

Protein from Animals and Legumes

beans with cheese
chili with beans

For best nutrition, choose rice that is brown, pasta that is whole wheat or made from Jerusalem artichokes, and bread that is whole grain. As a general rule: the darker the color, the more nutritious it is.

Checklist for a
Slimming—and Healthy!—Diet

- Eat more whole grains and fruits and vegetables.

- Do not eat (or drastically cut back the amount you eat of) refined and other processed sugars and any foods high in sugar content. Read the package label; ingredients are listed in order of quantity.

- Eat fewer foods high in total fat and partially replace saturated fats with polyunsaturated fats.

- Cut down on animal fat and choose poultry, fish, and lean red meats with a lower fat content. Prepare dishes that do not use a great deal of meat; for four, a half pound of meat prepared with grains and vegetables is adequate.

- Except for young children, substitute low-fat and nonfat milk for whole milk, and low-fat dairy products.

- Decrease consumption of butterfat, eggs, and other high-cholesterol items.

- Decrease salt consumption. Processed foods are often high in salt; fast foods are even higher.

Fiber, That Fabulous Low-Cal,
Low-Fat Filler That's Actually a
"Diet" Food

If you are eating the amount of complex carbohydrates we suggest, you are probably getting an adequate amount of fiber in your diet. Not only will you reduce your chances of getting a number of diseases Western people are especially prone to, research has shown that your body will actually absorb fewer calories! Remember those rats at the University of Virginia? A friend of ours became a vegetarian—with a little fudging—a few years back, but without a thought in the world of losing weight. Meals of wok-cooked vegetables with brown rice became common. The result? Minus 10 pounds. Since meat is the high-calorie item on most folks' plates, calories were cut inadvertently.

To make you feel good about all those ailments you are less likely to get if you have adequate roughage in your diet, here they are: appendicitis, diverticulitis, polyps, hemorrhoids, hiatus hernia, varicose veins, artherosclerosis, and ischemic heart disease. Perhaps the biggest bonus of adequate roughage is that the risk of certain intestinal cancers appears to be reduced. The length of time potential carcinogens are in contact with the gut wall is greatly reduced because increased fiber speeds up stool traveling through the intestines.

• Fiber is found in vegetables, fruits, and grains that have escaped the refiners—whole-meal wheat, rye, and oats. Whole-grain breads, oatmeal, brown rice, and bran are especially good sources.

• Vegetables with a high fiber content are cabbage, beetroot, carrots, broccoli, tomatoes, Brussels sprouts, eggplant, squash, parsnips, cauliflower, green peas, and lima beans.

• Among the fruits, look to apples, citrus fruits, and berries. The type of fiber found in apples, grapes, and oranges (pectin) appears to effectively reduce fat and cholesterol in the blood.

• Don't forget the nuts and seeds. Instead of peanuts, why not munch on unsalted sunflower seeds—they contain practically everything you need, including good-quality protein. But enough is enough. They have calories too.

Miller's Bran

• If you are still constipated—even slightly—you might add one teaspoon to three tablespoons of unprocessed, or miller's, bran to your food. Sprinkle it on your cereal, stir it into soups and stews, add it to pancake batter, dust it on salads. Bran has the highest fiber content of all foods.

● Before you buy a loaf of "bran" bread, check the ingredients. Wood pulp is added to some to increase the fiber content. There's nothing wrong with eating wood pulp—but why bother? Whole-grain breads are high in fiber without extras. "Ham on pine" perhaps?

● Don't go overboard with the bran. Start by adding a teaspoon a day to your diet; add more if you need it. You'll know when you're getting enough. Too much in the diet impairs the body's ability to absorb iron, calcium, zinc, copper, magnesium and possibly other minerals. Adding bran to a diet that is otherwise nutritionally poor may be worse than not adding it at all.

● If your diet has been largely meat, eggs, high-fat foods, and refined carbohydrates, proceed slowly. You might feel bloated if you eat too much fiber all of a sudden—and your stomach will rumble. Increase your fiber foods gradually.

Starve and Stuff?

While some people seemingly do well on the "starve and stuff" regimen of a single meal a day, usually at night, be aware that the one-meal-a-day eating pattern greatly increases the body's ability to make fat and will make losing weight harder. A recent study comparing four different eating patterns found that those who divided their calories throughout the day lost more weight than those who consumed them all at the same meal, even though the amount of calories was exactly the same: 1,000.

One group ate a 250-calorie breakfast, a 250-calorie lunch, and a 500-calorie dinner; their average loss was two pounds a week. Another group skipped breakfast, had a 250-calorie lunch and a 500-calorie dinner. They should have lost more weight, right? Wrong. Their loss was also approximately two pounds a week. A third group had only a 500-calorie meal each day, meaning they consumed exactly 3,500 less calories per week than the group who had three meals a day. Yet they didn't lose any more than the first group, which had three meals a day!

And the "starve and stuff" set, the ones who had a generous 1,000-calorie meal each day, and nothing else? *They lost less than a pound a week.* Obviously, the body is most efficient when it receives small quantities of food at regular intervals. Keeps you from feeling hungry, too, and so you're less likely to gorge yourself.

Planning Slimming Meals (and Snacks)

You know what you shouldn't eat, we'll wager, and here's what you should be eating:

- One vegetable salad per day. Two would be better.

- Two pieces of fruit per day—three if you are well within the day's calorie total. Save them for snacks.

- One or two slices of whole-grain bread per day. Or bran muffins.

- No more than four eggs per week.

- Fish two or three times a week.

- Other meat (beef, pork, lamb, chicken . . .) two or three times a week.

- Organ meat, especially liver, once a week.

- Whole-grain cereal (varied) three or four times a week.

- A glass of skimmed milk, cultured buttermilk, or yogurt each day. It counts if you put it in your coffee or tea.

- A starchy vegetable once a day (potatoes, dried beans, turnips, parsnips, lima beans, pumpkin, corn, peas, and so on).

- Two vegetables per day in addition to the salad and starchy vegetable.

- Eight glasses of water per day. Carbonated water, mineral water, and herb tea may be substituted.

17 Thin Tips for Taste Thrills

or, How to Be a Thin Gourmet

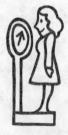

Thin cooking is different from fat cooking. Naturally, you say "Food isn't going to taste the same anymore because I won't be able to pour butter over everything—and all those cream sauces I love so. . . ." Oh, woe is you, nothing will ever taste good again. You'll lose weight because the food is so *blah;* you won't want to eat.

Wrong. You have a surprise in store for you. Food will taste as it never tasted before because you will be savoring the natural flavors and textures that got lost under rich sauces previously. And with imagination and a little know-how, you can prepare feasts so delicious that no one will suspect that they are low in calories too!

In the last few years some of the most celebrated food writers in America have lost weight under doctor's orders. These people have to work with food every day. They dream up new recipes, try out old ones, plan menus, write up food columns. They shop for food far more often than we do. They have people in to enjoy the fruits of their labor—truly—and they dine at restaurants often. Their whole working day is spent with something we are trying to help you not focus on; yet they have lost weight.

One of the first things they did was learn how to cook food *so that it wouldn't be fattening.* The food had to be agreeable in color, texture, and taste, just as it was before, but it had to help— not hinder—their weight-loss program. Craig Claiborne, a friend of ours, turned his physician-mandated reducing program into a tremendous success: His diet gourmet cookbook became a best seller. Obviously, he didn't do that by publishing a lot of recipes that lacked appeal. If you like to cook, you should add one or more of these new cookbooks to your collection; your family and friends will never know they're eating "diet" fare.

But even without new special recipes, there are many tips to shortcut the calories and turn your meals into special events that would please any gourmet.

• Learn to cook with less salt—or none at all. (See box on page 74.) We get all the sodium we need because it is contained naturally in many foods. In addition to the fact that salt is a leading cause of high blood pressure (and if you lower your intake of salt, your blood pressure will usually follow), it helps us to retain water, keeping us puffy and bloated.

• Fish is delicious broiled with chives, pepper, paprika, lemon juice, and a touch of tarragon, if you like the taste. Thin fillets will be done in a few minutes. You don't want them to dry out, but to retain their natural juices. You won't even miss the butter.

• Poach your fish. White wine, either alone or diluted with water and seasoned, makes the dish both elegant and low calorie. Diet food?

• Cut up carrots, onion, celery, green pepper—any vegetable actually will do—cover with water and poach the fish on top. Takes anywhere from eight to twelve minutes. As soon as the fish is flaky, it's done.

〜〜〜〜〜〜〜〜〜〜〜〜〜〜〜〜〜〜〜〜〜〜〜〜〜〜〜〜〜〜〜

Cutting Back on Salt

- Make your own fresh mustard from dry mustard powder, water, and herbs—dill and tarragon are good choices.

- Season green vegetables with lemon juice and oregano. If you don't have lemon juice, a bit of apple cider vinegar will do the trick.

- Fresh horseradish is great with cold salads, hot fish, and lots of other things. Try it—you'll be surprised at the pungent bite it adds.

- Vinegar and dill or basil are good with tomatoes, cucumbers, sliced cold zucchini wedges.

- If you don't already have a pepper mill, buy one. Try freshly ground pepper on nearly anything you used to salt before.

- Be sparing with cayenne—it's hot!—but it adds zest to fish, veal, chicken, and casseroles.

- Use scallions, shallots, leeks, garlic, onions, and chives in your salads.

- Do not use cooking wines—they contain a great deal of salt. Any table wine will do fine. And you get flavor, not calories, since the alcohol burns off during the cooking.

〜〜〜〜〜〜〜〜〜〜〜〜〜〜〜〜〜〜〜〜〜〜〜〜〜〜〜〜〜〜〜

- And you can broil fish without butter.

- A chicken roasted with several cloves of garlic will be plenty flavorful—without any salt at all. Here's how: Rub the chicken with a garlic bud. Pop one in the cavity. Put one each where the legs meet the breast. Stick bits in the wings. Put a few pieces on top. Roast for ten minutes at 400° F; turn down to 350°. Your chicken will be done in about an hour.

• You can do exactly the same with slices of fresh ginger. The chicken will have a slightly tangy taste.

~~~~~~

Some Calories Are More Fattening than Others

A calorie is a calorie is a calorie—right? Wrong. Certain foods, although they have the same number of calories as others, are more likely to put weight on you, according to a Maryland researcher, Dr. Richard Passwater. He claims that although a jelly doughnut and a four-ounce hamburger contain the same number of calories (250), the doughnut is twice as fattening as the hamburger, since it contains a large number of grams of simple carbohydrates (not the nutritionally sound complex carbohydrates), which will produce more fat.

Simple carbohydrates, the kind that won't do you much good, are found in junk food: cakes, pies, white bread, cookies, potato chips—anything that is overrefined.

Some doctors say that even on 1,000 calories a day, you will gain weight—if you are consuming lots of junk foods.

~~~~~~

• Use cornstarch or arrowroot for a thickener. Although they have the same number of calories as flour, you only need half as much.

• A word here about cooking in quantity, a scheme that works for some people. Preparing meals in large batches and freezing what you are not going to eat immediately saves time and *keeps you out of the kitchen*. You can plan your meals easily because you know what's in the freezer. You can approximate your servings to suit you—not the supermarket or the butcher. You can save money frequently since you are buying in quantity. You can take advantage of sales. And you will cut down on time preparing food, a vulnerable time for most people who habitually overeat. A taste of this, a spoonful of that, a snack because it's there—it all happens in the kitchen.

• In the winter, you can have steaming, thick soups and stews. Foods like yellow pea soup, stews with a zillion vegetables and a touch of meat, boiled chicken with rice and vegetables, nearly anything that can be cooked in a single pot. Usually there's enough for six or eight people—or a week's worth of dinners. Not only would it be boring to eat the same dish all week, it wouldn't be nutritionally sound because it's best to vary foods, remember? The solution: Immediately freeze a half or more in separate containers. That way you have meals ready and waiting in the freezer. You don't overeat because it's not just a leftover, it's another meal.

• *Discover Chinese cooking. It takes just a bit of oil to stir-fry meats* and vegetables.

• Buy a stainless steel vegetable steamer and steam vegetables. Or sauté them in a wok with a tiny bit of oil. But no matter what method you use, only cook them until barely tender. They'll be brighter, crunchier, and will have retained a goodly amount of their vitamins and minerals. When you overcook, more than half of the nutrients evaporate.

• To get your broccoli stalks done at the same time as the florets, cut stems halfway up the stalk. And don't forget to try broccoli raw—it's great in salads or with a dip.

• Iron skillets work nearly as well as the "no-stick" pots and pans, and you may be ingesting minute amounts of Teflon. You do get a bit of iron when you cook in cast-iron pots, but it's good for you.

• Sauté onions and mushrooms in a little soy sauce.

● Don't think you're doing yourself a favor by sweetening with molasses or honey—they contain simple sugar, as does white granulated sugar. And honey and molasses contain more calories than sugar. Brown sugar is no better either.

● Use instant broth instead of oil or butter if you can. To reduce the saltiness, dilute with twice the amount of water.

● You can have mashed potatoes. But instead of using butter and milk, whip them with skim milk, chicken broth, yogurt, or buttermilk.

● Try these on baked potatoes: slivered pimento and green pepper; a spoonful of stewed tomatoes; coarsely ground black pepper; dill; toasted sesame seeds; buttermilk, yogurt, or low-fat cottage cheese whipped with lemon juice in a blender.

The *nouvelle cuisine* of France can make diet eating a gourmet treat. Try these and see:

● Cook *all food* as little as possible to preserve flavor, texture, and nutrients.

● Instead of using flour as a thickener for sauce, rely on puréed vegetables, particularly onions, mushrooms, fennel, and leeks. Boil the vegetables in a little broth or water until barely tender, then whir smooth in a blender, adding broth as necessary.

● When sautéing, use no more than a tablespoon of butter. Poach chicken and seafood in broth or clam juice.

● Instead of cheese for an appetizer (which is traditionally a dessert), serve *crudités*—raw carrots, broccoli, cucumber slices, asparagus, cauliflower, celery, scallions, green pepper, zucchini, radishes, nearly anything goes—with a yogurt-based dip. Curry is yummy.

● Cook pasta made of whole wheat (only 155 calories per cup) and serve with finely chopped fresh tomatoes, barely steamed broccoli, and slivers of wilted green and red peppers, all spiced with herbs.

Lowering the Boom on Fat

Now since there's no way you're going to eliminate all the fat in your diet, your plan of action should be to cut down wherever and whenever you can. The overall rule is to try to substitute polyunsaturates for saturates; that means, vegetable oils for butters and margarines.

- When making soups from fatty meats or poultry, make them ahead of time, let them cool, and skim off the fat that rises to the top.

- Substitute skim milk for whole milk in recipes. Or use half whole milk, half skim. Use milk instead of cream. In some recipes, unsweetened fruit juice can be substituted for milk altogether.

- Choose lean ground round or chuck instead of the fattier ground meats. If the meat seems too lean and dry for your taste, add a smidgen of vegetable oil or grated raw potato.

- Substitute two-thirds of a cup of polyunsaturated oil for every cup of solid shortening or butter called for in a recipe.

- When a recipe calls for eggs, use two egg whites for one whole egg. This won't work in recipes calling for a large number of eggs but will work fine in those calling for one or two eggs.

- Substitute yogurt for sour cream. Since yogurt liquefies easily, add carefully and do not stir, beat, or heat too much. Yogurt gives dips a pleasant tart taste.

- Do not think you are getting ahead of the game by using imitation dairy products. Ban them from your life. Most of them contain the most saturated of all oils—coconut. It usually doesn't mention this on the label, and will only be listed as "pure vegetable oil." Coconut oil is the one usually used in nondairy creamers, ᴀᴧᴧᴧᴧᴧᴧᴧᴧᴧᴧᴧᴧᴧᴧᴧᴧᴧᴧᴧᴧᴧᴧᴧᴧᴧᴧᴧᴧᴧᴧᴧᴧᴧᴧᴧᴧᴧ

How to Lower Cholesterol with Food

Eat two grapefruits a day to lower serum cholesterol levels, suggests a scientist at the University of Florida. Pectin, the dietary fiber found in citrus fruits, and especially the type of pectin found in grapefruits, is thought to inhibit absorption of cholesterol in the blood. Its high content of methoxyl may be the protective factor. Although not promising a positive lowering of cholesterol, the doctor suggests that the amount of pectin in two grapefruits might do the trick.

Best way to eat a grapefruit: Peel it like an orange. That white stuff that sticks to the peel is loaded with bioflavonoids, one of the complex ingredients in natural vitamin C.

Or eat oatmeal a few times a week. Scientists at Rutgers University have found that eating a normal portion of oatmeal three or four times a week prevents the cholesterol in foods like eggs from being absorbed.

Other foods that help lower cholesterol are apples, oranges, celery, any whole-grain cereals, mushrooms, and cauliflower.

ᴀᴧᴧᴧᴧᴧᴧᴧᴧᴧᴧᴧᴧᴧᴧᴧᴧᴧᴧᴧᴧᴧᴧᴧᴧᴧᴧᴧᴧᴧᴧᴧᴧᴧᴧᴧᴧ

cheaper margarines, artificial sour cream, and most processed foods.

● Chicken skin is high in both fat and calories. Skin that piece before eating. And, just as with most people, younger and smaller birds are leaner.

● For a tasty salad dressing, mix yogurt or buttermilk with mayonnaise; add spices and herbs if desired.

● Eat ice milk rather than ice cream, and you'll get only half the fat of ice cream.

• Remember that "hydrogenated" on a label indicates that a normally unsaturated fat has been saturated with extra hydrogen atoms. You may think you are getting a polyunsaturate, but you're not.

• Trim the fat from your meat with shears. Gives better control and you can cut closer.

18 Booze

or, What More Needs to Be Said?

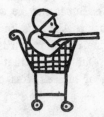

If club soda or orange juice is your drink, you can skip this section. But if you're like most of us, you prefer stronger stuff. And it's here many a dieter has gone awry: Alcohol is not only dangerous to your driving, but also to your diet. Drinks do not satisfy your craving for food; in fact, quite the opposite is true. Cocktails usually stimulate appetite. Sure, drinks can relax you, but they usually relax your willpower at the same time.

• Hard spirits (Scotch, bourbon, vodka, gin) are 75 calories an ounce. Most bartenders pour drinks that are more than that, especially at private parties.

• A four-ounce glass of wine contains between 75 and 100 calories. A spritzer even less. Naturally, the more soda and less wine, the fewer the calories. You can have three of these in an evening and only total around 200 calories. Ask for club soda with a splash of wine and a twist of lemon.

• Eggnog is a no-no.

● Gin, rum, and liqueurs should be *verboten*. Gin (made from juniper berries) has an adverse effect on the central nervous system, and seems to cause intoxication quickly; rum is high in sugar and calories, and so are liqueurs.

● But cook with wine if you want to. Not only will the touch add flair to your meals, the alcohol and calories burn off during the cooking. But use regular 25-calorie-an-ounce wine, not the dessert or "cooking" wines, which have more calories.

● Stay away from mixers like Coke, ginger ale, and tonic water. The calorie count of a drink goes up, natch.

● The higher the proof, the higher the amount of calories. Eighty proof liquors have 100 calories per jigger (ounce and a half); 90 proof, 110; 100 proof, 125. A lot for a little. But it may be what you need in order to not feel sorry for yourself. Also, it's known that people who have a glass or two of wine or other spirits in moderation are less prone to heart disease. Our guess is that the person who drinks a bit is less demanding of himself, less of a rigid perfectionist, than the teetotaler.

⁂

Lifesavers

Even if you weigh only 15 pounds more than average weight for your height and build, your life expectancy could be reduced by as much as four years.

19 The Cocktail Party

or, There's More to a Hangover than a Headache

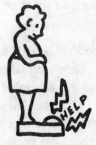

- If you ask your hostess for a diet beverage or a club soda and she doesn't have it, tell her that this happens often and you have some in your car. She wouldn't mind if you drank that, would she?

- Scientists have found that people who drink gallons of diet beverages really do not lose that much more weight than people who reduce without them. Probably that's because while the soda satisfies your oral gratification at the time, it doesn't do anything for the sugar craving—and the person finds a way to fulfill that later on. Sure, he's not drinking cherry soda, but he is stuffing down a secret package of cupcakes to get that same high. So drink your diet soda if you must, but if you are still not satisfied, why bother? You may be better off having a tiny portion of your sweet passion and getting that out of the way.

- A better choice at a cocktail party, and one that the bartender is sure to have, is club soda with a slice of lime or lemon. No one can tell that's it not a real drink, and it tastes more like one than a diet soda.

- Arrive late. It's fashionable. It's less fattening.

- See that tempting dish of peanuts? Don't have a single one. It makes not having a handful possible. Four ounces of peanuts doesn't sound like much, but they add up to 780 calories—which could amount to half your daily intake!

- Don't eat the whole hors d'oeuvre. Nibble off the top, stuff the rest into a napkin.

- If it's a buffet, check out the whole spread before you choose. Hot dishes usually have lots of fattening sauces, so try to stick to cold meats, salad, and fresh fruit.

- Pick the harder cheeses (Jarlsberg, cheddar, Swiss) rather than the creamy Bries or Camemberts. Hard cheese contains less butterfat and may be eaten without crackers. But remember that hard cheese has about 50 calories per ounce, a bit high for someone who's trying to lose weight. If you're going to make it dinner, that's okay, but keep track of the total. Spreadable cheese has about 80 calories per ounce, and then there's whatever you spread it on.

- Forget chips and pretzels. A single chip has 10 to 15 calories and is high in fat and salt content. Besides, they're addictive. Ditto for pretzels.

- Eat before you go. If it's a big cocktail bash, having something at home first makes it easier to pass up those calorie-laden hors d'oeuvres. Rolls of salami stuffed with cream cheese. Bacon wrapped around water chestnuts. Mounds of chicken liver pâté, bean dip, creamy salmon spreads. Baskets of attractive crackers, loaded with salt. Wedges of every imaginable kind of cheese, and they are all your favorites. Baby quiches.

- Look for the crudités—the colorful plates of sliced vegetables that have managed to become popular today. Dig in, but chew slowly.

• If you feel you must have one or a few of the other foods being offered, tell yourself exactly how many beforehand. That way you'll be able to pick and choose, knowing that you selected what appealed to you most. And you won't feel so guilty about going off your plan that you'll be tempted to have a half dozen more, because what difference does it make? Plenty.

• Just before you feel your hand start quaking as the tray of hot canapés comes your way, say to yourself: "A moment on the lips, an inch on the hips." Say it once, say it again, say it until you feel as if it has always been your credo. Eventually, it will be.

• Okay. Say you fail. At this party, you went completely on a binge—eating just like the old you—and when it comes time to put down all the food you ate it goes something like this: four Scotches; a handful of peanuts—no, two handfuls; three melted cheese and crabmeat canapés; a hunk of Brie; several crackers; a piece of Jarlsberg and that other cheese I never had before; half a dozen olives; quiche (baby); half a dozen Swedish meatballs; two shrimps; and, because I know it's okay to eat vegetables, lots of carrots and celery and broccoli dipped in the blue cheese gunk. That was before dinner. By the time you have written this all out, you are hating yourself. You may have already stepped on the scale and seen that you have gained an unbelievable five pounds! You want to die! You think what a terrible person you are, that you have no self-control, that this is as it's always been in the past, and so forth. STOP. Realize that, yes, you did go on a binge, you put yourself on "automatic eat" rather than staying in command, but then forgive yourself. After all, you haven't committed a felony. You have only let yourself down—temporarily. Look at to-morrow as a new beginning, and promise yourself that next time you will be better prepared mentally to have a night on the town.

Don't feel you have to abandon your whole plan simply because you transgressed for a night; see the matter in its proper perspective and move on. If every time anyone made a mistake he simply gave up and never tried again, the world would be a sorry place indeed.

So, forgive and forget. But resolve to be better next time. And once you are, the time after that will be a whole lot easier. You will have proved to yourself that eating thin is possible, no matter what's set in front of you.

20 How to Survive the Holidays

or, But I'll Die if I Can't Pig Out on Plum Pudding

Nearly everyone has trouble controlling weight during the holidays. You have not been singled out—even the size 6 across the room has to watch it during the annual high season of social gatherings. It seems as if everyone who has been thinking about having a party in the last year decides to do so in the few weeks between Thanksgiving and January 15 or thereabouts. What's a body to do? Without feeling deprived? Plenty. Remember that you are in control of your life. How you feel, what you do, what you put into your mouth—happens because you will it, not because the outside events overcome you.

- Eat only the foods you like best at each party. Why bother with the rest?

- Think of party eating like a banking transaction. If you overdraw tonight, "pay back" tomorrow by cutting down your daily calorie allowance.

• For starters, tell yourself that it's only *this once* that you have to get through the season (or day) without going off the diet. Next year, you will be thin and a few liberties will be allowed. And remind yourself that your goal is more important than the food of the day.

• When you are going to a cocktail party, don't go on an empty stomach. Have some yogurt, an apple—even an open-faced peanut butter and banana sandwich—before you go. That way you'll be less tempted by the plates of hors d'oeuvres.

• Skip the eggnog, after-dinner liqueurs, or mixed drinks and stay with white wine or brandy neat. For cocktails, stay with Scotch, vodka, or bourbon straight or with water or club soda.

• Before you walk in the door, have in mind how many drinks you are going to have, how many canapés—and stick to it!

• If you know that you are likely to be depressed during the holiday season, don't sit at home and brood because no one is calling you to come over. You call them. Plan a meal—if you aren't up to cooking a whole dinner by yourself, make it a potluck affair. You'll probably find more friends that you anticipated without something special to do. But do not wait until 3 P.M. Christmas Eve to start making plans.

• Plan activities for the day. Instead of simply sitting around all day with your family, why not go caroling? It will burn off calories and take your mind off food. If you live in an area where you can go ice skating or tobogganing, so much the better. The kids will love it.

• Keep the TV off. It will only encourage you to stay glued to the chair, hour after hour. Chances are you'll keep on snacking.

• Take normal (or tiny) portions of everything you want to eat. Just because it is Thanksgiving doesn't mean that you should have three helpings of everything. Your waistline certainly doesn't know the difference. But don't skip something you especially want (even if you only have a teaspoon), or you will end up feeling deprived.

• Somebody else gives you more food than you want? Douse it—discreetly of course—with black pepper. Or hide it under a lettuce leaf.

• What if you can't hide the leftovers on your plate? Cut them into tiny pieces and move them toward the edges of the plate. It will *look* as if you've been eating.

• Be polite—but remember to say "No, I couldn't eat another bite." Thin people have this sentence in their repertoire, and so should you.

• If you are the one who has to prepare the meal—let's say on Thanksgiving—why not ask for help from others this year? How about if you do the turkey and they do the vegetables and desserts? Tasting a little of this, a little of that—it all adds up and *should go into your food diary*. But if others help, you won't be putting as much temptation in your way. Think you can't ask? How would you react if someone asked you for help and told you why? Of course you would do what you could. Besides, it's time to start speaking up for your needs. If you can't find someone to take over a part of the preparation, get somebody in the kitchen to help you, someone who knows what you are doing. They will keep you from tasting everything in sight; they can taste for you.

• And prepare foods with less sugar and fat than the traditional recipes you've used in the past. Sweet potatoes do not need brown sugar or marshmallows. Mashed potatoes do not need a quarter of a pound of butter. Use whole-grain bread when stuffing the bird. For new recipes, check the magazines. Many will have reduced-calorie recipes that are just as tasty as those overladen with sugar and fat.

• Give leftovers to guests as they leave.

• Don't buy lots of candy for the children. Not only will you help them to not have the same fat-fighting problem you have, you won't be tempted to eat it if it's not around. Keep fruits and nuts on display.

• Don't give food as presents. Have you always made relishes and jams for house gifts? Not anymore. We want to get you out of the kitchen!

• If someone gives you food for a present, give it to someone else *right away*. The kids down the block—or your thin neighbor—will love you.

• If you are going to stay with family or friends for a few days, stock the fridge with low-calorie snacks for yourself—and of course you'll share. Ask for a tiny space to keep your edibles. Even the most insensitive hostess will come around once she sees how serious you are.

• NEVER LET YOURSELF GET RAVENOUS. YOU'LL OVEREAT AT THE NEXT MEAL.

• Pass up the pies. Pecan has nearly 500 calories in a single piece, minced meat, 350. Fruit pies are better, and if you have to sample one, eat just the filling and leave the bottom crust; you'll save 75 calories. But don't have the plum pudding. Tell yourself it is the holiday season and you'll get another chance at it later in the week.

• Go to all the family affairs and dinners—don't punish yourself needlessly. If the array of food is overwhelming, yet it is somehow important to the hostess and you that you taste everything, do just that. Taste. A teaspoon (or good heavens, a whole tablespoon!) will satisfy your desire to have a little of this, a little of that. Remember that everything must go into your food diary.

• Tell yourself that if you come out of the holidays weighing the same as when they began, you deserve a pat on the back. An actual loss would be even more spectacular, but don't fret if this doesn't happen.

• And if you do eat more than you wish you had (and who

doesn't), don't berate yourself and tell yourself it's hopeless, you are a lowlife, you will never lose weight, and so on. Just put it behind you and get going again. Nothing really worth achieving is ever simple.

21 Restaurant Dining

or, What Am I Doing in a Place Like This?

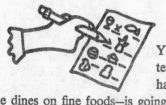 Your first visit to a restaurant after you begin your new eating behavior—especially the type where one dines on fine foods—is going to be, well, at least an interesting experience. Just as at home you have certain learned behaviors, you have a different set of patterns that emerge when you are in a restaurant. Do you always order the complete meal instead of a la carte because it's a bargain? That way you get an appetizer and dessert for only a dollar or two more than the price of the entree, right? Do your eyes always wander down to the dessert column while you are still deciding between prime rib of beef or scallops in sherry sauce? Do you always start a meal with an appetizer? If you answered yes to all of the above, rest assured that you have plenty of company all around the world.

But now you are going to take a new tack, because you have decided to live life differently. Dining out can be just as pleasurable as it was before, but you can walk away without feeling stuffed. If the business lunch is *de rigueur* for you, don't despair. Of course you can use your new behavior at the best restaurants in town; in fact, often the pricier the place is, the more willing they will be to accommodate you.

• Plan ahead. If you can, select the restaurant, or type of restaurant. One where you know you can get plain broiled fish and a salad. One where you will be able to ask for a combination of vegetables that isn't on the menu.

• If it's a lunch that will be somewhere in the vicinity of your office, pick a place that is a brisk fifteen-minute walk to and from it. Allow yourself enough time so you won't be tempted to step into the street and say "Taxi!" Look upon the walk as a treat to yourself, a bit of exercise that fits into your day easily. Window shop, look at the people in the street, and try to leave the problems of the office back there. Or work out a problem that doesn't seem to have an easy solution.

If you pick a restaurant a half mile away from your office, you will cover a mile a day if you walk both ways. That's a hundred calories you wouldn't have burned if you rode in a car or slipped into the place next door. If you were to do it three times a week, you would drop roughly five pounds a year.

• If you have decided in advance what you want, order without seeing the menu. Nearly everyplace has some sort of broiled fish— or you can ask that it be done plain, without butter, with lemon and spices—and some sort of tossed salad. Don't tempt yourself needlessly by reading over all those rich dishes you aren't going to order.

• Ask that the bread be removed entirely from the table, if you can, or place it next to your companion's plate. Ditto to the butter dish.

• If you don't want the baked potato or the rice or whatever that your entree comes with, speak up. And if the waiter brings it just the same, ask him to have it removed. Remember that you are the diner, and the servers are there to serve you.

• If you feel obligated to join your companion in a cocktail, be aware of calorie differences. A glass of white wine has half the calories of hard liquor. A spritzer—a combination of white wine and club soda—naturally has less. And today with so many executives weight-conscious, it will not seem at all unusual if you switch from a martini to a white wine. Look around the room. You may have never noticed it before, but look at all those grown men sipping glasses of white wine.

• Better yet: Ask for Perrier or some other bottled water. It will usually be brought to you in a glass of ice with a twist of lime. It looks classy and is refreshing to the palate. Again, you are in good company. Some of the most high-powered men and women dining around the room made the switch long ago. Calories: *zero*.

• If you feel you must order an appetizer, choose clear soup, tomato juice, or a fresh fruit cup. It will keep you busy while others are eating pâté on toast.

• Always avoid casseroles or dishes with sauces, unless you can have the sauce on the side. That way you can elect to eat most of the dish plain or with just a smidgen of the sauce.

• Order dishes that must be eaten slowly. Half a cold lobster, and just bring lemon instead of mayonnaise, please. We're not going to take you through the menu because if you are serious about this plan, you are well aware of what is laden with calories, what is not. Remember, the simpler the dish, probably the fewer the calories.

• Eat slowly and leave a lot on your plate. If your companion notices, say something like "Oh, I'm just not hungry today." He has no reason to doubt you.

• When it comes time for dessert, instead of saying "No, thanks" or "I'm not having dessert, but go ahead," simply tell the waiter you are having coffee for dessert. Your client may then be less self-conscious about ordering a peach melba. Or you can have fruit. Plain. Hold the cream, whipped or otherwise. Strawberries are nearly always available in most good restaurants and a portion will have only about 50 calories.

• Frequent the same restaurant. The captain and waiters will get to know you, and know that you do not want the bread, you like your fish plain, the salad should be brought without the dressing, and so on. They will anticipate your special requests and not think you are strange.

- There is another way of dealing with restaurants, but it works best with a friend who isn't a client. Decide beforehand that you are going to have a half of a tomato, sliced, cucumbers, lettuce or spinach, a hard-boiled egg, carrot slices, whatever, and ask the waiter to have the salad made up special for you. Tell him that you can eat only certain foods—bring up your mysterious allergies. Carol Channing—who does have allergies—is known for bringing her own food to restaurants when she joins others.

- If you are staying at a hotel for a few days and will be dining there, ask to speak to the chef about your special needs. Ask that your fish and meats be broiled without adding butter; the vegetables cooked with spices and herbs but no fancy sauces. Once the chef understands that you are serious about your regimen, he—and your waiter—will most likely take you under their wings and try to make your meals delicious and satisfying—without lots of unnecessary calories.

- Be the last person at your table to start eating.

- *Eat slowly.* Just because you are paying to have your meal prepared does not mean that you must eat every single bite. If the waiter checks to see if you have finished before you think you have, stop and think for a moment: Am I still hungry? Am I full? You may have passed the satiation point without realizing it. One of the biggest problems fat people have is realizing when they are full.

- When you have finished, give yourself—and the waiter—a signal. Place your fork, tines up, at an angle across your plate. Fold your napkin next to your plate. And NO NIBBLING.

- If you know the restaurant is famous for something, and you know you will be unsatisfied unless you have a taste—go ahead. There is a chain of hamburger restaurants in New York that has the best piccalilli anywhere, according to one of the authors. She knows it's loaded with sugar. And she always has some when she is there. But if it's not great, why bother?

• When eating out, why use up calories on food that you can have every day or prepare for yourself? Or dishes the restaurant prepares poorly. Enjoy the best—you deserve it.

Eating French

• For an appetizer, have an artichoke. Eating it will take at least twenty minutes and you'll get only 150 to 200 calories if you go *very* easy on the butter or vinaigrette. Pass on the hollandaise.

• Mussels vinaigrette is another good choice. Less than 100 calories.

• Avoid: anything prepared *rémoulade,* which means with a mayonnaise dressing; onion soup made with cheese and bread; vichyssoise and other cream-based soups.

• For your main course try rack of lamb, which is trimmed of fat before roasting. A better choice than lamb chops, which are not.

• Fish is usually available a number of ways. Pass up those with rich sauces and order instead: *sole véronique* (smothered with grapes), anything poached or served *à la nage.* Mussels *marinière,* steamed in a white wine sauce, looks huge, is low in calories, and takes forever to consume.

• Fresh fruit in season is a good choice for dessert. Strawberries. Raspberries. *Très chic.* Or *crème caramel*—it's not as bad as an éclair.

Eating Chinese

• Chinese spareribs are cooked exceptionally lean. You could make them a main course.

• The soups are fine as long as you don't overindulge on the fried noodles.

• Avoid: anything fried—egg rolls, shrimp, rice. Plain rice is okay, as it has only 100 calories per half cup.

• Ask that the chef hold the MSG, salt, and sugar, and go easy on the oil. In most establishments, they will be glad to comply, since there are a number of spices used in Chinese cooking.

• Gourmet treat: whole steamed fish in black bean or ginger sauce. Enough to share with a companion, whether or not he or she is dieting.

Steakhouse

• Suggest somewhere else!

• A small piece of prime sirloin (two by three inches, an inch thick) amounts to 350 calories, lots of fat. So eat small and give the rest to your companion to take home in a doggy bag.

• Have a double shrimp cocktail as a main course.

• Or broiled shrimps. Nix to the Fried Fish Platter.

• Pass up the fries and onion rings. Order the redoubtable baked potato, season with a sprinkling of freshly ground pepper.

Eating Italian

• Order the antipasto as a main course. There is usually enough to make anyone happy.

• If it's pasta or die, see if it's available with a vegetable sauce. Le Cirque, one of the toniest places in Manhattan, specializes in it, and it's not listed on the menu. Those who know, know. Ask for *primavera* with pasta.

• Shrimp scampi is not too bad, but it is loaded with oil so eat with caution.

• Anything *piccata* will be sauteed plain with lemon. Pass on parmigiana.

• You do not eat garlic bread. It is addictive.

• For dessert, try zabaglione. Although it tastes fattening as can be, it's a whipped egg and sugar concoction spiked with Marsala and has only about 200 calories a serving.

Eating Mexican

• Stick to a tostada with vegetables; stay clear of the tacos and enchiladas.

• Plain corn tortillas with chile sauce are fine for nibbling. Avoid the corn chips that are already on the table—high in fat and calories.

Eating Japanese

• Sushi and sashimi (raw fish) are excellent. So is steamed fish and any dish with lots of vegetables and little meat.

• Leave the tempura for another time.

Seafood

• If you are going to order shellfish, watch your cholesterol for a few days before or after, since all shellfish (lobster, shrimp, clams, oysters, and so forth) are extremely high in cholesterol.

• Stay away from anything dipped in batter and deep fried.

• Order fish broiled plain or "dry," baked, or poached.

• Ask the waiter not to bring tartar sauce and to hold the butter. If a dish comes smothered with a sauce, scrape it off and season with pepper and lemon.

Restaurants with Salad Bars

• Pile up on the raw vegetables and be wary of the pickled or canned items such as beets and beans, since they contain sugar and salt. Pass by the bacon bits, olives, and pickles.

• Choose the greens that are the darkest in color since they contain more vitamins than the pale ones. Iceberg lettuce may not have many calories, but it hardly has nutritional value at all.

• Forget the high-fat, creamy dressings. Use vinaigrette or lemon juice. Unless a dressing is specified as yogurt or buttermilk, assume the creaminess comes from mayonnaise.

• And there are those who would say to avoid restaurants completely for the first week or two of a diet.

⌁⌁

Caffeine Blues

There's no way around the fact that caffeine is not good for you, and especially during a diet. When the body burns fat for energy, you may find it hard to sleep and your hands may shake. Eliminate all caffeine and try taking two aspirins or acetaminophen (Tylenol) before retiring—unless your physician says you shouldn't.

If you must have that coffee taste on the palate before you end a meal, at least try decaffeinated coffee and tea. Perhaps, for a change, try herbal tea. Now there are some who say even decaf isn't good for you because the processing to make it that way may be carcinogenic. Look for the steam-process decaffeinated—nutritionists say it's okay.

⌁⌁

22 Eating in a Coffee Shop

or, The World Is Full of Potholes

One of the worst possible places in the world to look for nutritious and low-calorie food is a fast-food emporium or a coffee shop. Try to avoid the fast-food places altogether. Or save them for an occasional visit and "treat" if you can't stand the thought of going without a Big Mac this month. Step inside the door, and immediately you will conjure up the combination you have had in the past. Perhaps you had a Big Mac, French fries, and a vanilla shake. Just a normal, satisfying meal, right? Wrong. That cost you 1,094 calories—maybe your whole day's allowance.

Coffee shops are somewhat easier to handle, since there are usually items like salad and plain tuna that you can order. But remember, you must always plan in advance and stick to your guns. Here's a list of food usually available in most coffee shops that will allow you to lunch or brunch without overloading:

- Order your sandwich open-faced. Not only will you eliminate a slice of bread (60 calories or so) from your daily intake, cutting the sandwich with a knife or fork will take longer. You may not feel the need to finish the whole sandwich. Remember, if you are concerned about starving children in the world, give to UNICEF.

Food	Calories
Dry cereal in a box	70
Skimmed milk (four ounces)	40
Whole milk (four ounces)	75
Egg cooked without butter	75
Cottage cheese (two tablespoons)	25
Tossed salad (no dressing)	30–40
Two slices of tomato	15
Cantaloupe	50
Apple	70
Small can of tuna, drained or water packed	150

• Skip the house dressing. It's usually oil and vinegar. Lemon juice and garlic, pepper, and onion make a fine dressing. After a while, you'll wonder how you could have eaten salad bogged down in oil. Picture pouring straight oil down your throat.

• See ordering a low-calorie and satisfying meal in a coffee shop as a challenge. And see yourself as a winner when you walk out the door.

• If you usually lunch in a coffee shop, consider bringing your own lunch to work. The low-calorie treats you can prepare at home will make that smoky, crowded joint seem just what it is. Vegetable salads with cottage cheese, nutritious soups in a thermos, fruit combinations, hard-boiled eggs, shrimp, cold sliced chicken, or turkey; the list can be as long as your imagination. Not only will you save calories, but money also. After you eat, there will be plenty of time to do errands or just go for a walk.

23 The Cafeteria Clutch

or, Why Do They Put the Desserts First?

One way to get around the prospect of facing the baked lasagna and chocolate cream pie that cafeterias seem to favor is to ask a friend to get your meal. She won't have any trouble resisting the calorie-laden goodies for you; but that's just a stopgap measure for those days when you know you can't face the choices on the cafeteria line, whether it's a college dorm or the company lunchroom. But there are ways to go down calorie lane without courting disaster:

• Avoid casseroles. Even if the choice is between a casserole and something fried, the casserole will almost always have more calories.

• Nix to butter. Nix to white bread.

• Keep your entree as dry as possible. No, you do not want gravy or sauce. No, you do not need tartar sauce. But a wedge of lemon (harboring near the tea) will spice up nearly everything.

• Some days, pass on the entree and have just vegetables. Try for at least four servings of vegetables a day.

• Have two or three fresh fruits a day. Take the fruit at lunch or dinner but save it for a snack later.

• Go through the line with a buddy. If your friend is also dieting, so much the better.

• Join the line after the desserts if they come first. Why make yourself be strong when you can avoid the temptation entirely?

• Put each piece of food on a separate plate. Your tray will fill up and you won't feel deprived. Or tempted to take a dessert.

• Take your tray back as soon as you have finished eating. It will signal that the meal is over.

• For a main-course dish that tastes like a dessert, take a fresh fruit and a container of plain yogurt and mix.

• And if you will simply die unless you have a sweet dessert, take Jell-O. It will have fewer calories than the other sugary choices.

24 Snacking

or, Will I Ever Be Able to Eat Anything Gooey Again?

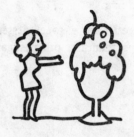

Lots of people do not have a hard time consuming sensible meals; they eat no more than anyone else —perhaps even less—at breakfast, lunch, and dinner. But it's what happens the rest of the day that does them in. Perhaps you can't resist the coffee cart once you hear the familiar bell ring. Or maybe you munch while you are cleaning house. A cookie here, a cookie there—who's to notice? Perhaps you nibble in bed while you wend your way through the latest thriller.

Once you start keeping records, your food diary will make you aware of such automatic eating, which has nothing to do with hunger, and that in itself can be the first stop to shifting from automatic gear to manual—*where you must think about every bite you take.*

If you find you are snacking throughout the day, there are probably any number of people, places, and events that trigger the eating. You may not be able to eliminate all the food cues you have gotten used to through the years. For example, the coffee cart is going to come every morning, like it or not—but there are ways to sabotage food cues so that they no longer control you. You are in charge here, remember?

Eventually, the food cues will no longer bring on an eating response, and your only thought when one of them crosses your path will be an occasional memory of how you used to react before.

And this doesn't have to mean that anything gooey, sticky, creamy, salty, or sweet will never cross your lips again. It will if you want it to. But less often. And less of it.

• If you usually have a Danish at midmorning and a doughnut midafternoon when the coffee cart comes along, take a walk to the bathroom instead. Check your makeup or brush your teeth or wash your hands.

• If you must have coffee, have someone else get it for you. Take them into your confidence about why you are avoiding the coffee cart yourself. Otherwise you'll be branded uppity.

• But try to cut down or out on coffee anyway. Just like sugar, it causes your energy level to yo-yo; which—surprise—stimulates appetite.

• Plain popcorn makes a fine snack. As long as it's *plain*.

• Have an apple and eat it *s-l-o-w-l-y*.

• Plan to have snacks. If you know that your energy sags at 4 P.M., have some food ready for a hunger attack, but make it something good for you: an apple, an orange, half a banana. At home, keep your refrigerator stocked with carrot sticks, radishes, parsnips, cauliflower, celery, fresh coconut, fresh pineapple. And keep them out front so they are the first things you see when you are "just checking" the refrigerator.

• Take a plastic Baggie with low-calorie snack items to work. When others have a Danish, you have half an apple or carrot sticks.

• Remember to record the snack in your food diary. Count the calories in your daily allowance. THIS IS IMPORTANT, if you are serious about losing weight.

• If you are at home, eat every snack off a plate. (Since it will seem odd if you pull out china and silverware to have an apple at the office, you can forgo this away from home.) What you are aiming for is to lessen the number of food cues in your life, and making a slight production of eating snacks will help.

• It will also make you ask the question: Do I really want to bother? Am I really hungry? You want to eat when you are hungry—and not just when the idea strikes you.

• Before you have the snack, have a glass of water. Many times the water will make you feel full and do away with the craving for calories. Good for the skin, too.

• If there is a snack food you HAVE TO HAVE EVERY NOW AND THEN—let's say it's a Twinkie—don't tell yourself that you will never be able to let it pass your lips again. You'll feel deprived and sorry for yourself—and reach for a Twinkie. Work it into your diet, say, once every two weeks, or have half as much. (Once every other day is obviously cheating, and you know it.) Eventually, surprise of surprises, the food you couldn't do without will lose its appeal as your tastes change. And you'll wonder how you ever ate it with such abandon.

• DO NOT KEEP JUNK FOOD AROUND THE HOUSE. Just because you always kept ice cream in the freezer before—in case unexpected company dropped in—doesn't mean you have to go on doing it. How often was that ice cream really consumed by "company"?

• If your diary notes that you almost always eat forbidden foods alone, make a pact with yourself that you will only eat in front of other people. A chocolate bar consumed in front of someone else goes a lot further than one you secretly stuff down while you are grocery shopping. Of course, this only works if you do not live alone. A goldfish doesn't count.

• Remember that Twinkie? Go ahead—have it. But only in your mind. Imagine your way through every single bite.

• Great for spreading on crackers: cottage cheese or a combination of farmer cheese and yogurt whipped in a blender with garlic, pepper, lemon juice, soy sauce, and herbs—tarragon, oregano, chives, basil, parsley, thyme, rosemary—any combination or a pinch of each.

• When you go to the movies, decide in advance if you are going to eat anything—don't wait until you are walking by the candy counter. Remind yourself that whatever passes your lips must be entered in your food diary, the calories figured into your daily total. Tell yourself how bad sugar is for your metabolism—how it will briefly satiate you, then make you crave more. And if you must have something, remember that popcorn—unbuttered, naturally—is an ideal snack. Two cups of popcorn, cooked with oil and salt but without extra butter—averages about 80 calories and provides bulk in your diet, making you feel full and satisfied.

• If you like nuts, buy them in their shells. Not only will they be salt free, you'll consume fewer because you have to bother shelling them.

• Although the commercials make them seem like everybody's favorite diet aid, diet sodas are not necessarily going to help you lose weight. True, if you have been consuming regular soda and switch to diet, you will cut down on calories. But it has been proven that people who constantly sip on diet soda lose no more weight than those who do not. Besides, many contain caffeine, that old appetite stimulant.

• When you reach for that first peanut, tell yourself that you are only going to have one or ten and stick to that. Keep reminding yourself that just because you have a single peanut, you have not blown the whole diet, or even the day. You are in charge here.

• If watching television is a food cue, try knitting or crocheting instead. Or hooking a rug or wood carving.

• If it's something sinful you're hankering for, wait ten minutes. Ask yourself if you really have to have it.

25 At the Halfway Point

or, Where You've Been and Where You're Going

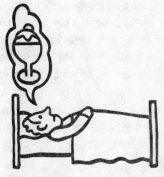

One of the easiest ways to get depressed when you are dieting is to not have anyone notice that you have already lost 20 or 30 pounds. "Here I have been working so hard, and not a single person has noticed." You feel sorry for yourself, and wonder if it has been worth it—after all, somebody must see that you're thinner! Well, if you are wearing the same clothes as before, it is difficult to notice that you're wallowing around in them these days, that they are hanging looser. But put something on that fits and—presto!—the world can see you are thinner *right now*.

Obviously, you can't afford a whole new wardrobe every time you go down a size, but a small investment here and there may make or break your whole diet. In addition, it is important to start learning to live with the new you, to make adjustments in the way you see yourself and the way others see you as you go along. Then you won't be at such a loss dealing with the new you.

So, do invest some money. Get your clothes altered along the way. Buy a new dress or a suit that fits. The reinforcement that it will give you is well worth the price.

- Why not try out other beauty and grooming routines that appeal to you but you denied yourself since you were "too fat"? Try a new hairstyle. Maybe you would like to try a new color, too. Sure, everybody will notice, and instead of feeling self-conscious, take the attention and compliments (don't count on them, but don't think they are phony either) with grace. Just like a thin person.

- When your size 20s are too big for you and can't be altered to fit, give them away. You are never going to need them again. If you keep them around, if you hang on to your old clothes just in case you get fat again, you are striking an unconscious bargain with yourself: One day I will be fat again. You are committing yourself to failure. And when the 16s fall from you, give them away. And so on. The symbolism attached to getting rid of clothes that no longer fit is a positive reinforcement that this time, indeed, you are making a change for life. Besides, the idea that you will have to go out and buy a whole new wardrobe should you gain 20 pounds will help keep you slim.

- Examine any "fat" habits that you might have and see if you still need them. Are you afraid to sit on chairs that don't look strong enough? Maybe they weren't when you weighed 305. But now? Do you unconsciously turn sideways going through tight places? Do you still need to? Get rid of these habits as you go along. The point is to not be overwhelmed by everything when you reach your goal.

- Have you always wanted to play tennis or badminton, to disco dance, or swim, but felt too foolish doing it when you were carrying around all that weight? Now is the time to learn. Sign up for lessons three months down the road, when your body is thinner and all the walking or whatever you have been doing has it in shape. Looking forward to lessons you have always wanted can be a powerful impetus to losing weight.

• Stop thinking about what you don't deserve and what you do. Most fat people unconsciously tell themselves that "as long as I'm fat I don't deserve better." Perhaps the particular area of conflict is a job, or your family, or a relationship with someone of the opposite sex. You may have gotten used to accepting less than you deserve. It's time to reexamine the major areas in your life and see if you are indeed happy with the way things are. Are you taken for granted by your coworkers, your boss, your spouse or lover, your friends? Are you the genial, always happy "fat" person that nobody really knows? Now it's time for a change. You have been working so hard at changing yourself physically, you probably haven't given too much thought to how you should be changing psychologically. Sit down, give yourself quiet moments of reflection and talk to yourself about what you want out of life and how you are going to get it.

You no longer need to feel at a disadvantage at the bargaining table at work because the other guy is thin. You deserve—and must demand of yourself—equal treatment, equal respect. Unless you start speaking up for the person you have always wanted to be, you will be at a constant disadvantage and extremely vulnerable to putting the weight back on.

It's the same with many people who have ever had what they perceive to be a defect. We know one woman in her thirties who once had a rather large nose. It was so big, in fact, that when she was twelve the boys called her "Big Nose!" She never quite recovered emotionally from that experience, even though in her early twenties she finally went ahead and had a nose job. She still saw herself as a person with a big nose who wasn't quite entitled to a good relationship with someone of the opposite sex. If any man came along who treated her well, her unconscious reaction was that something must be wrong with him. She only stayed in relationships where she got a raw deal. Her friends kept after her, though, and finally she was able to work out those old feelings and find someone who treated her as she deserved.

It is the same if you are carrying around a distorted body image. If you become obese as a child or adolescent, you will have a more difficult time shedding that image—like the woman who couldn't see herself without her old nose. *But if you want the weight loss to remain, you don't have a chance unless you can change your image of yourself.* You need to work just as hard at this as losing the actual pounds or you are bound to gain back what you have lost. You have to learn to match the fantasy of being thin with the reality. Therapy, enrolling in a behavior-modification program, reading, and introspection all can help. It will take time and new experiences to implement what you are telling yourself about the new you. But until your new self-esteem feels like a second skin, you are in constant danger of backsliding toward the baklava.

● Indulge your vanity. As a fat person, you probably thought it was ridiculous to spend too much time thinking about what you would wear, how you would do your hair, what kind of makeup was "in," and so on. It's the same for men. Sure, you may have thought it's fine for thin people to be self-absorbed about how they look but absurd for fat old me. It's time to learn that it is okay to pamper yourself. At first it will feel odd, but everything feels strange with something new. You may have always thought you couldn't go in and try on clothes without buying anything. Phooey! Everyone does it. And you need to start seeing yourself in new clothes, brighter colors, seeing how they look, and also finding out what it feels like not to be obligated to every single person who gives you the time of day. Sales clerks are used to browsers. So go shopping even if you don't have a cent in your pockets and your credit cards are at home. Buy fashion magazines that you never read before. You might not want to wear the way-out fashions, but they'll give you ideas to help you change your image.

But a note of warning. Realize that a lot of thin people have the same fears and insecurities that you do. Does everybody seem to turn and stare as you walk through the door of the local pizza parlor or disco? Realize that it isn't just you. They look at *everybody* who comes through the door. Just watch.

Not every single dream can come true just because you are thin.

If you have told yourself for years that everything would be absolute bliss if only you were thin, you are in for a big letdown. No one's life is an endless string of good times and emotions. Unless you prepare yourself for the fact that life is at best a bumpy road for everyone, slim and fat, you are likely to be disappointed and not see the point of continuing the diet or maintaining your weight. So while it is all right to have expectations, temper them with reality. An old friend of ours—a reformed alcoholic—said the other day, "You can't either despair or hope. All you can do is take one day at a time. And help usually comes from the most unexpected sources."

And last but not least: Always keep your eye on the goal.

〰〰〰〰〰〰〰〰〰〰〰〰〰〰〰〰〰〰〰〰〰〰〰〰〰〰〰

Dealing with the Dragon

Mouth dry? Do you have bad breath? Or is that a fruity taste? Not pleasant, but it means that your body chemistry is changing. An occasional antacid can help by neutralizing stomach acids. Look for one without sugar. A caution, however—calcium antacids should be used very sparingly unless you have a minimum of calcium in your diet. Calcium may be absorbed and deposited in the tissues with too much use. Look instead for antacids containing magnesium or aluminum, which are not absorbed.

〰〰〰〰〰〰〰〰〰〰〰〰〰〰〰〰〰〰〰〰〰〰〰〰〰〰〰

26 Exercise

or, Taking the Bus May Be Dangerous to Your Health

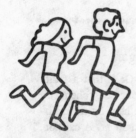

You knew this was coming. Maybe you skipped right past it the first time you skimmed the book, but here it is again, refusing to go away. Your reaction might be: Oh, my God—they're going to ask me to exercise! And you're thinking: Nuts to them. I won't! I can't! I'm embarrassed! I read somewhere that actually dieting is the only way to lose weight—you have to exercise hard for an hour to burn up as many calories as there are in a single piece of apple pie!

True. But what if you exercised and didn't eat the apple pie—you'd be way ahead of the game, wouldn't you? And what if you exercised like that three times a week?

Although it used to be thought that exercise played only a small part in weight reduction, in the last few years we've learned that one of the major differences between obese and thin people is *the amount they exercise*. Often the two groups of people will not differ in amount of calories consumed, but in how many are burned off by activity during the day.

In children this is especially marked, since one survey found that overweight girls and boys may actually consume several hundred fewer calories per day than their leaner peers. But the overweight group spends only a third as much time each day in physical activities as the normal-weight group.

wwwwwwwwwwwwwwwwwwwwwwwwwwwwwwwwwwwwwwwww

Did You Know . . .

that exercise not only burns up calories during the workout, it perks up your metabolism so that you continue to burn more calories for the next few hours?

that although dieting peels off the pounds, it can't firm and reshape your body?

that the more overweight you are, the more calories you will burn during any activity? It takes energy—calories—to move a mountain.

that disco dancing can burn up as much as 450 calories an hour?

that a fifteen-minute walk every day will burn off 2 pounds a year?

that you should exercise as much as you can in the outdoors without eyeglasses, contacts, or sunglasses so that unadulterated sunlight can reach your eyes? Full-spectrum light—whether the sun is shining or not—appears to tune our body clocks and keep us healthier.

wwwwwwwwwwwwwwwwwwwwwwwwwwwwwwwwwwwwwwwww

Among adults, the same is true. Swimmers and joggers (no, we don't mean professional athletes, just normal folk who swim and jog) actually consume about 600 calories more a day than do sedentary types of the same age and height; yet sedentary men and women weigh between 20 and 30 percent more.

And it appears that the reason we gain weight as we get older is primarily related to the fact that while we may not be eating more, nearly all of us are less active and *consistently* burn fewer calories during the course of the day. The word consistently is significant, for it is this continuous decline of calories needed that makes the pounds creep up month after month, year after year. We tend to slow down when we get married, and become more sedentary as we get older, and this begins happening somewhere in our twenties.

If we decrease energy expenditure by only 100 calories a day—let's say a half hour of easy bicycle riding—and do not accordingly decrease food intake—we are likely to gain somewhere in the vicinity of seven pounds a year. The number would be somewhat higher were it not for the fact that it takes calories to maintain extra poundage, even when it is just sitting there. That's why heavy people burn more calories during exercise than thin individuals.

It is generally believed that we consume fewer calories than our grandparents did, yet more of us today fight the battle of the bulge. And once again, the main difference appears to be our sedentary life style. It's brushing with an electric toothbrush, shining shoes with a gadget you switch on, grinding coffee beans in an electric grinder, opening a can of tuna with an electric can opener, washing and drying clothes in "automatic" machines, cutting the turkey with an electric knife. It's riding the bus to work rather than walking, and complaining because the bus stop is two blocks away. It's riding the elevator to the third floor. It's driving the car around the corner rather than walking. With all these labor-saving gadgets around, we have to make the extra effort to see that they don't become our own worst enemies. Just as we read to cultivate our minds, so should we walk the extra mile for our bodies.

What all this means is that exercise and activity—regular and frequent—can play a major part in not gaining weight, lowering weight, and keeping it off. We tend to think of diets as having a beginning and an end, and usually we make no particular changes in our life style other than eating less for the duration. But for a lifetime of being slim, vigorous exercise and regular activity must be incorporated into our daily routine.

Now that we've given you that little sermonette, we have plenty of up-to-the-minute scientific data on why you should exercise.

Read them over those times when you just don't feel like exercising.

Why Exercise?

• *Exercise decreases appetite.* That old myth about feeling hungry and eating more after exercising is just that—a myth. Of course, we are not talking about leading a dog team to the North Pole. We are talking about the amount of exercise you get from a half hour of jogging or an hour on the squash court. And it's more than simply a matter of "Now that I have burned off X calories, I don't want to eat and put them all back on," even though that is naturally a part of what is going on. Why you feel that way in the first place has at least two physiological explanations.

The body is "tuned" best when it gets a normal amount of activity. When you are in good shape—or finely tuned—your body efficiently regulates appetite (and calorie intake) to match calorie burnoff. Physiologically, the body knows that what comes in should be expended, and vice versa. A mechanism in the brain called the hypothalamus has among its jobs the regulation of appetite. When it doesn't get any activity signals, it's at a loss as to exactly how much food it should suggest the body needs. This is obviously simplified, but in general it's one of the ways the hypothalamus works.

Another theory takes this one step further. The hypothalamus, just like a thermostat in your home, responds to fluctuations in heat. Exercise warms the muscles, which stokes the internal body temperature, which in turn informs the hypothalamus that it need not switch to the "hungry now" position. When it's hot outside, your furnace doesn't need to run, does it? It gets by without extra fuel. So do you. This theory also explains why we are likely to eat less (some of us, anyway) in the good old summertime. If you've never noticed that salads that don't satisfy in January seem quite filling in July, you aren't listening to the beat of your internal drummer. The body is quite an amazing machine, knowing what's good for it and what's not. Like your mother used to say, "If you would only listen. . . ."

• *A certain minimum amount of exercise per week is needed to reduce the risk of heart attack.*

The more you exercise, the more this risk is decreased. This is especially important if there is a history of heart disease in your family. A big stack of studies, including one with nearly 17,000 Harvard graduates, showed that the more physically active you are, the lower your risk of suffering a heart attack. There are a number of reasons for this. A body that is in shape is better able to distribute oxygen to the tissues, thereby increasing their capacity to work. Many people, especially older folks, have a heart attack immediately after they've shoveled the driveway after the first heavy snow of the winter. Perhaps it was the only hard physical activity in a year; the body couldn't handle it.

And a heart that's been exercised pumps more blood with each stroke, so it *never* has to work as hard.

Oxygen to the heart itself is increased because the whole network of tiny blood vessels feeding into the heart is larger in an active person, as are the openings of the coronary arteries.

Physically active people have lower blood pressure and fewer irregularities in heart rhythm, both of which are related to heart disease and stroke. More and more doctors these days are putting their patients on exercise programs as a way of reducing blood pressure, sometimes with drugs, sometimes without.

What else does exercise do? Plenty:

• *Helps control cholesterol.* Several recent studies show that active people have higher levels of a blood protein known as HDL, which carries away cholesterol instead of letting it clog up arteries.

• *Reduces anxiety and stress.* Vigorous workouts for at least thirty minutes three times a week dramatically alleviate depression. Jogging seems to have the greatest effect, possibly because after about fifteen minutes of exertion, the brain releases morphine-like compounds called endorphins that produce a "high" in the brain's pleasure centers. Some doctors now routinely prescribe exercise when treating depression.

The sports that have the greatest effect on mood are those that work up a good sweat and increase heart rate for at least fifteen minutes at a time. Suggested: swimming, bicycle riding, jogging, and walking at a fast pace; tennis isn't bad, but not as good as those listed above.

And it's worth noting that even individuals who don't think they're depressed start feeling better once they get regular exercise.

• *Relieves premenstrual blahs.* An excess buildup of water—along with the salt it retains—may be the reason for the blues in the days preceding a menstrual period. Sweating during a workout gets rid of some excess water and salt.

• *Keeps varicose veins in check.* Continuous, rhythmic, and repetitive exercise keeps the blood in the veins flowing rather than stagnating. When the blood is flowing easily in time with the heart, the veins will stay as small and flat as possible. Check first with a doctor to be sure there are no blood clots already trapped in varicose veins before a vigorous workout.

• *Improves complexion.* That healthy glow is caused by increased circulation, dilation of surface blood vessels, and a lessening of nervous tension.

• *Cures insomnia.* When muscles are tired, you'll have no trouble falling asleep.

• *Reduces the risk of osteoporosis,* or the loss of bone strength that usually comes with age, especially in women. The bones' ability to absorb calcium, which they need for strength, is enhanced by frequent workouts.

• *Controls the side effects of diabetes.* Diabetics often have blood that can be called "sticky," and that is likely to clot; regular exercise reduces this risk and makes the individual more sensitive to insulin, possibly allowing the dosage to be lowered in time. Obviously, don't do this by yourself—get a medical opinion.

• *Promotes a sense of well-being, enhances ego,* dissipates anger, resolves frustration, and relieves boredom. When you are feeling dragged down and out at the end of a day, what you may need is actually a good workout rather than a nap or that cup of coffee. Exercise is so good for you, in fact, that unless we stop now it will begin to sound like snake oil.

Increased Activity, or Squirm Your Way to Thinness

Just jumping around more during the day will obviously use up more calories than if you sit like an immovable mass. We are talking about little ways to increase physical activity in your daily routine, ways that may seem a bit odd at first, but should eventually become a part of your life. Remember that if you have ever been heavier than you are right now, you have more fat cells than a person who's been forever thin, and so you have to keep those guys in check. Here are sneaky ways to do it—the sneaky part is that you will hardly think of them as exercise. It won't seem at all like the dreary calisthenics you've been dreading we'll recommend.

• Wiggle around in your seat. Tap your feet, shift your weight around. Use your hands for emphasis when you talk. Cross your legs. Uncross them. We don't mean you should turn into a Nervous Nellie who can't ever sit still, but people who do squirm a bit use up about 25 more calories per hour than those who sit still. Why bother, you say? Well, because if you do it every day for a year, that extra energy expended amounts to 18,250 calories. More than five pounds.

• Clean your house. Vacuum your rugs. Often. Look upon housecleaning not as a boring chore, but as a chance to get a workout. For the 120-pound woman, cleaning expends between 150 and 250 calories per hour. And if you push that vacuum cleaner harder—and faster—the aerobic benefits increase accordingly.

• Answer the telephone farthest from where you are. If you are downstairs, use the upstairs extension, or vice versa. We know this seems extreme, but it works.

• Ditto with the bathroom.

• Whenever you can, climb stairs rather than ride the elevator or escalator. After four flights, you start giving your body a cardiovascular workout—not to mention the calories burned. If you can, do two steps at once, using only the railing for balance, if you must use it at all. It's good for the calves and thighs.

• If you work on the fortieth floor and aren't quite up to all that, ride up thirty-five flights, walk the last five. Do the same going down.

• Carry your own groceries rather than having them delivered.

• Park your car at the far end of the parking lot. If anybody asks you why, tell them it's less likely to be banged by someone else.

• Walk to work if you can. If you live in a big city, by foot is often the fastest route during the rush hour. Manhattan's Madison Avenue buses, between 5 and 6 P.M., can nearly always be beaten by the pedestrian.

• If you take the subway, get off a stop or two before your destination.

• If you walk more than a mile or so, start timing yourself. Getting the time down can be a game.

• When your electric can opener breaks, don't get it fixed. The energy you spend is power saved. There are probably other gadgets that do things for you that can be replaced with your own steam.

• Walk your clothes to the dry cleaner and back home again. Why let the delivery boy get all the exercise?

• Stand rather than sit. You will use up at least 10 more calories per hour. If you pace around, you expend almost a hundred more.

• Do leg lifts while you are on the telephone. Or just walk about. But always remember to hold the phone with your hand rather than cradle it with your jaw in the crook of your neck. If you do the latter, your jaw joint is likely to go out of alignment, and that can lead to all sorts of other problems.

• If you work at a desk, put the wastepaper basket across the room. Practice your shot. If you miss, get up, pick up the piece of paper, and deposit it each time you miss.

• If you work at a desk job (or if you are writing a diet book), get up every twenty to thirty minutes and stretch. Get a glass of water. Move your head around to release tension in the neck and shoulders.

• Exercise during the nightly news, or whenever. Stretch during the commercials.

• Get a dog. Great walking companion.

• Take the dog for a walk longer than usual. He won't complain.

• Play Frisbee with your kids. Or touch football, or take them skating.

• Plant a garden in the spring. Uses about 240 calories per hour.

• Stop using the drive-in window at the bank. Park your car and go inside.

• Instead of using your "in" and "out" boxes all the time, get up and walk to your secretary's desk.

• Instead of phoning your coworker when you want to discuss a point, walk over to his or her desk.

• Wash clothes often rather than wait until you've got a pile a mile high. If the laundry room is in the basement, you'll be going up and down more. Even if it's not, you'll use up more energy—of your own.

• Ask for a motel room on the second floor. For the view. Carry your own luggage if you can.

• Jump around when you blow-dry your hair. Bend over and stretch your hamstrings.

• Make love a lot.

In general, do chores for yourself. It may not seem as efficient or convenient as having everything done for you by someone else or a machine, but even a tiny expenditure of calories—done over and over again—will help you reach your goal of being thin. Take stairs. Go slowly, and you use 3 calories a minute; speed up the pace and the number jumps to 10 calories a minute. That's 600 calories in 60 minutes. If you climb stairs for only 10 minutes a day, that's 700 calories a week. Eventually, that adds up to nearly 10 pounds a year.

This business of how much you will lose and how much you will gain based on an exact counting of calories *in* and calories *out* is necessarily approximate. Because of the way our bodies work, we gain a pound for every 3,000 (actually a few less) calories consumed. This is because the new extra bulk contains water, and a pound appears on the scale before those calories actually tally up in total fat. However, when we lose, we have to eliminate water as well, which means we must shed nearly 4,000 calories, whether by diet or exercise—before we lose a single pound of fat.

Now when you are starting a weight-loss program, it's hard to imagine how great you will feel in a year when all that stair climbing pays off and those 10 pounds are gone. But remember that the year will go by with no help from you, and you could be 10 pounds closer to your ideal weight than you would be without climbing those stairs or scrubbing the floor. The increased activity will be especially important when your aim is to maintain your ideal weight. Those 10 pounds can offset approximately 140 martinis a year. It's not a bad bargain.

∿∿∿∿∿∿∿∿∿∿∿∿∿∿∿∿∿∿∿∿∿∿∿∿∿∿∿∿∿∿∿∿∿∿∿

R and R

Notice that on some days at the beginning of a workout you just don't seem to have the energy you had yesterday? Your body may need a day's rest to recuperate and rebuild, which can only happen when it has adequate rest. When you are up to twenty to thirty minutes per workout, you might give yourself a day of rest every third day to avoid chronic fatigue.

∿∿∿∿∿∿∿∿∿∿∿∿∿∿∿∿∿∿∿∿∿∿∿∿∿∿∿∿∿∿∿∿∿∿∿

Exercise: Which One?

Regular, vigorous exercise should be a part of everyone's routine. Period. This is how to achieve the most calorie burnoff. And the best way to reap the benefits we've outlined is through *aerobic* exercise, a form of movement that enhances the ability of your heart to pump oxygen to your limbs. For most fit individuals, this means raising the heart rate to more than 120 beats per minute for at least fifteen minutes three or four times a week. You can check this by feeling your pulse on the side of your wrist closer to your thumb (use fingers other than the thumb), or in your neck just to the side of your Adam's apple. Keep track for ten seconds and multiply by six.

⁕⁕⁕

Metabolic Magic

Once you manage to hold down your weight for at least two years, you may be one of those lucky people whose metabolism will start acting like a thin person's. You will not put on weight as quickly as you did when you were fat. Should you start to gain, the normal rate will be a pound a month—not four or five—which is a whole lot more manageable.

⁕⁕⁕

The key to success here is to choose a form of activity you enjoy. If you don't enjoy what you are doing, you won't continue. Sounds obvious, right? But many people force themselves into an exercise they really can't stand, just because it's trendy or what the neighbors are doing. Exercise, like your favorite color, is strictly a matter of personal preference. You may actually like the rhythmic measured routine of calisthenics, or it may seem no fun at all. Some of you will be bored if you can't exercise in the outdoors;

others will appreciate the feeling of gliding along in the warmish water of an indoor pool when it's 10° outside.

The point is, if you don't like what you're doing, you won't continue. Before you read about the different sports and what they can do for you, close your eyes and choose one or two types of vigorous activity that appeal to you the most. And that's what you should be doing three or four times a week.

We suggest two types of exercise because most sports develop only one set of muscles, and with a combination program, you'll be more likely to have all-over fitness. It's not overly muscular legs that you want but an all-over trimness. Some athletics, however, will work against each other, and so it's best to find two kinds of exercise that complement each other. Swimming and jogging are excellent, but weight lifting and swimming aren't. Working with weights tightens the muscles, while swimming relaxes them.

Naturally, before you plunge in, remember that vigorous exercise on a body that's not used to it can be dangerous. In general, anyone over thirty who has been sitting around for years should have a medical checkup before embarking on an exercise program. And regardless of age or previous activity, you should also check with your doctor if you have a chronic illness, such as diabetes, heart disease, or arthritis.

One more word of caution: Start slowly. Even though you may be bursting with enthusiasm, if you end up sore tomorrow, you aren't likely to repeat the process and your plans are likely to be forgotten. Also, your heart may not be able to handle too much too soon. A simple way to ensure that you are staying within your limits is to say a sentence out loud every few minutes. If you can't talk above a whisper without gasping for breath, *stop immediately*.

Walking

Although you won't burn off the calories the fastest if you go this route, walking is the easiest form of exercise for nearly everybody to incorporate into their lives. Now here we don't just mean the five-minute dash to the subway or supermarket: We mean walking briskly for at least a half hour, eventually working up to forty-five or sixty minutes a day, at least three times a week.

• In the beginning, the word is *caution*. Begin with fifteen-minute walks every day—or every other day. Stay with a pace that is comfortable for your condition. After two weeks, increase your walks to thirty minutes, gradually working up to forty-five to sixty minutes.

• Strive for regularity—otherwise you'll end up walking less rather than more. If an hour walk every other day is easier to fit into your schedule than a half hour walk every day, so be it. By the same token, fifteen minutes morning and evening (on the way to the bus, parking your car that far from work?) and thirty minutes another time bring nearly the same results as an hour's walk. But try to keep your walks at least fifteen minutes long—you need that much time to do any good for the heart, lungs, and so on.

• Although the aim is comfort and enjoyment, your pace makes a difference in the amount of calories you burn in a set time. The general rule is that you burn approximately 100 calories for each mile covered *on foot*. That means that if you do three miles an hour, you burn approximately 300 calories in that hour; at four miles an hour, you expend 400 calories. Four miles an hour is a very brisk pace, indeed, and you may not want to keep that up regularly.

• While you are walking for exercise, carry as few things as possible. Even a heavy handbag can make you feel exhausted and give you a backache if you walk for more than ten or fifteen minutes. In addition, you'll be lopsided and won't enjoy yourself as you should. Especially if you plan to walk to work, keep this in mind. Four pounds should be the limit for a handbag, no more than six for a briefcase.

• In most cities, twenty short blocks, eight long ones, or three times around a single block equals a mile.

• Walking may be one of the safest routes to fitness, especially if you are quite overweight and have been inactive for a long time. You didn't get fat overnight, and you don't have to walk it all off in a day.

- Ease your way into jogging (if you are so inclined) by alternating jogging with walking. Start by jogging a quarter of a mile, walking the next quarter, and so on until you build up your endurance.

- Some believe that walking is better exercise than jogging because your joints are spared the hammerlike effect of pounding the pavement. Ditto for the disks in the back and for the breasts.

- And others suggest that jogging ages the face since all that pounding causes the face muscles to sag.

- Wear sensible shoes, as mother used to say. Pinched toes do not a good or happy walker make. And to save your feet, adopt a heel–toe stride.

- Women might keep their high-heeled pumps at the office and walk to and from work in flats or jogging shoes.

- Suggested weekly workout: an hour a day at a brisk pace if possible, at least every other day.

Jogging

So much has been written about jogging in the last few years that we will keep it short and sweet.

- It is true. You will feel absolutely terrific once you work up to the point where you are doing somewhere between seven and ten miles a week. After about thirty minutes of jogging, those brain chemicals called endorphins, which produce a high in the brain's pleasure centers, are released. You'll feel euphoric under the shower and wonder why you don't do this more often.

- Although jogging has some perils, its pluses make it one of the best exercises for cardiovascular endurance, muscular strength, flexibility, balance, and muscle definition. It also aids digestion, sleep, and *weight control.* You'll expend between 10 and 13 calories per minute. Or somewhere between 600 and 800 calories an hour. A lot, in other words.

• On the minus side, jogging is hard on joints and ligaments. And if you become a fanatic, it is hard on lots of other things, including marriage. Somewhere we read that people who jog in the ten-mile-a-day range have one of the highest divorce rates around. Either that's because so much time and energy goes into making the run that there's not much left for anything else, or the jogger often adopts a new life style that eschews tobacco, alcohol, and other dissipations. Or finds another jogger.

• Get yourself into jogging shoes. The difference in the way you feel afterward will be nothing short of amazing. Buy shoes to suit the type of pavement or ground you will be striding across.

• If you are a woman, DO NOT JOG WITHOUT A BRA.

• Each stride while jogging uses up the same amount of calories as does a push-up. Now that's nice to know.

• It will take approximately ten minutes of jogging to work off a glass of beer; slow down to a walk, and it will take just about twice as much time.

• WARM UP BEFORE YOU TAKE OFF! And do more stretches when you quit. Warm-ups free the muscles and joints to perform fluidly; cool-downs relax the muscles and cool the body. And you'll be sorry if you don't do both. The main object is to put the principal body joints through their full range of motion. The exercises need not take longer than five or ten minutes.

• Some women claim that jogging during pregnancy reduces discomfort. Some women run in marathons during their pregnancies. Get medical approval before you do either, and *listen to your body.* Feel miserable? Quit. That goes for people who aren't pregnant and are of either sexual persuasion.

• Suggested weekly workout: a half hour at least three times a week.

Swimming

One of the things that is so terrific about swimming is that it's good for people of all ages, especially those over fifty. That's because the buoyancy of the water puts less stress on your joints than sports engaged in on land; even people with arthritis or orthopedic problems can sometimes move about freely in a pool.

• Swimming tones the upper body, flattens the stomach, develops the lungs, and helps tone the legs. It's especially good for arms and the pectoral muscles that hold up the breasts. And it's a great aerobic workout.

• Swimming is great for the head. Somehow it gets cleared out during a session.

• If the chlorine in the pool bothers you, try goggles. They can make swimming a lot more fun.

• The calorie burn-off is somewhere in the 350-to-450-per-hour range, depending on body weight and how strenuously you go at it. For instance, a 130-pound person working reasonably hard at the crawl will use about 450 calories per hour.

• Suggested weekly workout: twenty to thirty minutes, three to five times a week. Figure your distance so that you are doing at least five hundred yards. In a sixty-foot pool, that would amount to twenty-five laps.

Biking

Bicycle riding is the number-one choice for exercise among women, according to the 1980 Virginia Slims American Women's Opinion Poll. Roughly one in three women said she rides a bike— but she should know the difference between recreational riding (which is fine) and aerobic riding (which is what you want if this is one of your exercise choices).

For recreation, you can glide along on a ten-speed bike with very little effort. You may think that you've done enough in twenty minutes. But oh, no. To burn calories, you need to peddle against resistance. That old three-speed (or single speed) languishing in the back of the garage may be a better piece of equipment for your purposes.

• Bicycling correctly, for at least forty-five minutes a session and plugging along quite energetically, increases aerobic power and tones and shapes hips and legs. It doesn't do a great deal for your arms, but it does increase flexibility and gives you great quadriceps—those muscles in front of the thighs.

• Peddling a stationary bike—one in which the power is supplied by you, not the electric current—is an excellent aerobic exercise. Twenty to thirty minutes is enough, comparable to forty-five outdoors—since we tend to spend a lot of time coasting when the terrain pulls us along.

• Calorie expenditure again depends on how much you weigh and how hard you work. A 130-pounder going along at 5.5 miles per hour—which is on the slow side—uses up only 246 calories in an hour. If you weigh 25 pounds more and move along at 13 miles an hour—which isn't impossible—you more than double that total to 600 per hour.

• Suggested weekly workout: outdoors, forty-five minutes; stationary bicycle, twenty to thirty minutes; both, three to five times a week.

Aerobic Dancing

The focus is on fun and fitness rather than weight control, but your body doesn't care as long as it's burning away those pounds. If most types of exercise don't appeal to you—but you love dancing—this may be the answer. And once you've got the technique, you can do it at home to your own tunes. Slip into a sweatsuit or leotards and turn up the volume!

• It tones and shapes the entire body because all the muscles are used. And it increases aerobic power and flexibility. And gets you ready for the disco floor.

• Classes are offered in most cities and can be located through the Yellow Pages. Prices vary, with a series of lessons costing somewhere between $50 and $150, depending on location. Check your local school for evening classes; the cost could be even lower. Later, you're on your own if you want to be.

• Calorie burn-off is between 350 and 500 per hour.

• Suggested weekly workout: sixty minutes, two to four times a week.

Tennis

One of the side benefits of tennis is that tennis buffs always have something to talk about to others similarly inclined. Naturally, talking expends calories by moving the jaw up and down, and so you get that as a bonus if you take up tennis.

• If you are fit, tennis is good for all ages; best for those under forty-five. It is a good all-around toner, improves flexibility and balance, and strengthens arms.

• Calorie burn-off varies from 400 calories up to 600 an hour. Singles give a better workout than doubles, naturally.

• If you are going to use tennis as one of your "main" exercise programs, you should play three to four times a week; however, because it is an intermittent activity, combine it with one that has continual movement. Swimming, jogging, or skiing would be excellent.

Everything Else

• Cross-country skiing is probably the best all-around conditioning exercise there is. It builds endurance, exercises the arms and legs, promotes balance, and is absolutely great for weight control since you may burn up to a thousand calories in an hour.

• Downhill skiing may be full of thrills, but the calorie burn-off is much lower: 450 per hour.

• Calisthenics can burn up to 500 calories an hour, are great for shaping and toning and working at specific areas (thighs, hips, waist), but how many people do you know who do them regularly unless they are enrolled in a class or belong to a health club? Most people find them boring and although you may start out with great enthusiasm, after a few days (let alone a few weeks), calisthenics become somehow difficult to fit into your schedule. Something nearly always comes up. Unless you're one of those people who will stick with them, don't count on calisthenics to be your mainstay. You might find a few you like best—sit-ups are great because nearly everyone wants a flatter stomach—and work up to thirty or fifty once or twice a day. It won't kill you.

• Golf may be your game, and it is relaxing, but a great exercise it isn't. It has very little conditioning effect, especially if you ride around the course in one of those carts designed to keep you from walking. If you walk—and carry your own clubs—the benefits go up, but still it only uses up around 300 calories an hour.

• Bowling burns up about 172 calories an hour and is great for camaraderie—32 million Americans will attest to that. It is not an aerobic workout per se, but it does improve concentration and coordination. In combination with an aerobic exercise, it's a fine way to get more activity into your life. If you do take up bowling, also try to get an aerobic exercise three times a week.

• Basketball burns up about 500 calories an hour; it improves reflex response time in addition to providing a good all-around workout.

• Climbing stairs is an excellent exercise for both your weight and your heart. A person of normal weight can lose 6 pounds a year by simply climbing two flights of stairs per day; an overweight person can lose between 10 and 12 pounds. The average burn-off is in the 400 calorie-per-hour range. A British study showed that conductors of double-decker buses had substantially less heart disease than the drivers who merely sat. In the most severe form of heart disease—sudden death in early middle age—the conductors who did the climbing had only about a third as much as the drivers.

~~~~~~

Weighting Out the Winter

The average weight gain during the winter months is nearly 7.5 pounds, the result of stay-by-the-fire weather plus a change in eating habits. We suppose that extra layer of fat helps keep you warm, but if you would rather leave that up to your coat, make an extra effort to get more exercise during the frigid months. The good news is that exercising in low temperatures burns up calories quicker than in the warmer weather.

~~~~~~

Fitness Fables

• *Sugar just before exercising raises the energy level.* By the time that extra energy is realized, the tennis game is probably over and you've done nothing but send your body into the yo-yo effect of raising your blood sugar before it plummets. In some individuals, sugar just before a workout can do more harm than good. The only time you need to replace sugar is after an hour and a half of a hard and steady workout, such as a long tennis match or a cross-country race.

• *Take salt tablets to ward off fatigue.* Unless you are really sweating profusely, salt tablets will make things worse. They can cause nausea and vomiting. If you know that you will be sweating heavily during a regular workout, you might add a little extra salt to your diet; but most Americans get much more salt in their diets than they need anyway.

• *You need extra protein for extra strength.* Actually, excess protein is harder on the system—making the liver work harder, in-

creasing the need for water—than a well-balanced meal of carbohydrates and protein. Several studies show that high-carbohydrate
diets before exercising (or the night before a race) will increase
performance and stamina.

• *Don't drink while exercising.* Just the opposite. Drink as soon
as you are thirsty. When cells are dehydrated, your muscles lose
strength and your heart is under extra strain.

• *Don't eat spicy foods before exercising. Or gas-producing
foods.* Nonsense. So-called "forbidden" foods have no effect what-
soever on performance.

• *Take a cold shower after exercising.* The truth is, for winding
down after sports, nothing beats a tepid shower. Lukewarm water
dilates the blood vessels and cools the body, as well as relaxes the
muscles. A cold shower could cause a constriction of the blood
vessels in the heart as well as your skin. If you insist on having a
cold shower, start with tepid water and finish with cold.

27 Acupressure

or, Lend Me Your Ears

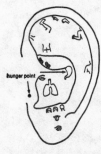

hunger point

Hungry? Give your ears a massage. The hunger pangs should stop in a moment or so. No matter how odd it sounds, many swear that it works.

Called acupressure (a cousin of acupuncture), the technique is based on the principle that by stimulating certain nerve endings, you will send your brain the message that you are full—no matter how hungry you felt a minute ago!

There are two methods. If the first doesn't work, try the second.

One: Insert your index finger gently into your ear orifices, with your palms toward your face. Put your thumbs on those little bumps of cartilage at the tops of the earlobes. Firmly massage the cartilage (tragus) with your thumbs and index fingers for one minute or more.

Two: Put your index fingers in the tiny depressions in front of and above your earlobes, just above the cartilage bumps. Massage for at least a minute.

L. D. tried acupuncture in the ears for appetite suppression. Tiny staples were placed just above the lobes. She was to twirl them when hunger struck. It seemed to work, but they kept falling out, and that necessitated extra visits to the acupuncturist, and finally she gave up. Apparently it works best if one's ears aren't pierced. Maybe that was the problem.

28 For Women Only

or, How Come We're On the Same Diet and He's Losing Twice as Fast?

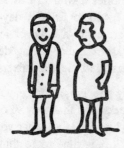

Ah, yes. You and your mate are on the exact same diet—you have even restricted your caloric intake more than he has by 400 calories . . . and yet, he's losing by leaps and bounds while you are s-l-o-w-l-y taking it off. Unfair! you want to scream. Go right ahead. It all has to do with making babies. In order to protect the fetus, nature blessed us with an all-over cushion of fat to provide protection and warmth. And no, it doesn't go away when we're not pregnant. It stays. It gives us curves and makes it harder for us to lose weight than men.

A woman's body has nearly twice the ratio of fat to muscle as a man's, and so it takes us nearly twice as long to burn calories and lose weight. Part of the reason is that fat needs considerably less energy to keep it happy and *there* than does muscle tissue. In addition, the female hormones—estrogen and progesterone—encourage our bodies to turn food into fat. Birth control pills give another boost to fat-producing substances and make us retain excess water. Do the cards sound as if they are all stacked against you if you are of the female gender? We suppose you could look at it that way. But since it's likely to remain that way until men start having babies, we figure you might as well know the facts instead of just getting depressed when you get on the scale.

• While an active average-sized man can lose weight on 2,000 to 2,400 calories per day, an average female must cut back to between 1,000 and 1,200 to lose. And that makes it difficult to get all the nutrients you need, which is why exercise is important to your health and well-being. Because the added exercise lets you consume more.

• Since 1930, according to a study conducted by the Campbell Soup Company, the average number of calories a woman can eat without gaining weight has dropped from 2,400 to 1,800 a day—equivalent to giving up a piece of chocolate cake, a bowl of ice cream, and a glass of white wine. The reason? Labor-saving devices such as dishwashers, vacuum cleaners, and electric mixers.

• Naturally, there is someplace (usually the hips) where you want to lose weight first. But it never works out that way. You lose it in the face and chest and arms, maybe—not at all what you had in mind. Fear not. Your body simply needs time to readjust and redistribute the remaining fat, a process that takes about a month. Exercise naturally helps. Regular, vigorous exercise helps to speed up the redistribution of your fatty tissue.

• On top of the fact that physiologically women have a harder time losing weight, in most households today it is still the female who is responsible for planning, buying, and preparing family meals, which means that women have to invest far more time, thought, and energy in food than men. Although it may not be possible to throw away the apron, you might ask your children and husband for help during the difficult weeks and months.

• When women are asked why they want to lose weight, they often say "to please my husband (doctor, mother, or children)"; men are more likely to say "because I want to look and feel better." Since it is always easiest to do something for yourself, think about why you want to lose weight—*think about yourself*. If you can talk yourself into wanting to please yourself with your new body, dieting will be a helluva lot easier.

• When you're tempted to go off your diet, sit down and list the reasons why. You should be able to poke holes in any "reasoning" you come up with and turn the slump into a time of renewed determination. We become strong because we have learned how to resist weakness.

• A large or sudden weight loss can interfere with your hormones and disrupt your menstrual cycle. Periods might be scanty or skipped entirely if you severely limit calorie intake. But the normal pattern should return once you're eating as a thin person normally would. If your period doesn't resume in a month or two, see a doctor.

• If you find that you are bruising easier during a diet, increase your intake of vitamin C and zinc, both of which will help counteract the effect of weakened capillaries. When the body is burning off its fat stores, excess estrogen may circulate in the bloodstream, and that makes capillaries fragile, liable to break, and bleed under the skin, which is seen as a bruise. Suggested dose: 500 to 1,500 milligrams of C; 25 to 50 milligrams of zinc.

• The food diary will make you aware of dietary patterns at different times of the month. Are you eating more sugar just prior to your period? That's not unusual, as the hormones make you susceptible to mood swings and depression. And it will probably be harder to keep up the weight loss during that time, too—you may even gain a few pounds (some women gain six or seven!) as your body retains water. As you record when you crave certain foods and when you gain, you will be relieved to know that biochemistry has a hand in weight loss and gain. You'll be less likely to go off your diet when you stop losing—if you know it's that time of the month. The weight will come off after your menstrual period. One way to curb the binge blues: B vitamins (a complex with at least 50 to 100 milligrams of most of the components) and eating complex carbohydrates.

29 Smoking versus Weight

or, I'll Get Fat if I Can't Have a Drag

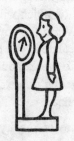 Statistics show that of those who quit smoking, a third will gain weight, a third will lose, and a third will stay the same. Even if you don't pop a chocolate bar into your mouth every time you want to inhale, there are reasons why you still might gain. Your metabolism changes; blood circulation improves and blood supply increases—some people will actually add up to two pounds of fluid due to increased blood supply. All of which will make you feel better, naturally, and should give you the energy to take care of the extra pounds with more exercise. But remember this: You have to exercise. It won't do any good to have the energy if you don't use it. In any event, once your body gets used to not having nicotine and tar coursing through the bloodstream, it will be fairly easy to shed those extra pounds. And there are other tried-and-true ways of keeping the lid on pounds and your hands off cigarettes:

• Drink lots of water. It keeps you busy, relieves tension, and cleans out your system, washing away the nicotine. And it can help avoid the constipation that sometimes accompanies giving up smoking.

• EAT THREE MEALS A DAY. This will help you avoid snacking and keep your blood sugar level regular so you won't be prone to a "down" in the middle of the morning and afternoon.

• The hardest time for some to not smoke will be right after a meal. Get up from the table immediately. Don't linger the way you did when you smoked. It might even help to give up that cup of coffee—you're probably used to having a cigarette with it, and by dispensing with the habit completely, it will be easier than going halfway. Go for a short walk instead—you'll be invigorated naturally, and the urge for the smoke will be gone for the moment. And you won't be tempted to eat the leftovers.

• Brush your teeth right after a meal. Your mouth will feel so clean, you can convince yourself you don't want to put anything as nasty as a cigarette into it.

• Take up knitting or needlepoint or crocheting. Busy hands don't have time to reach for the munchies. Fiddle with paper clips, worry beads, click pens if you must. Start working on a thousand-piece jigsaw puzzle. What you're after is something to divert your attention from the fact that you used to have a cigarette in your hands.

• Exercise. It helps release tension, and if you take up an aerobic sport—one in which deep, heavy breathing is involved—you won't want to foul up your ability with a cigarette. Swimming, jogging, and strenuous bicycle riding are all excellent.

• Increase your intake of natural sugar—the kind you get from fruits. When nicotine is withdrawn, your craving for sweets will increase temporarily, and satisfying that with natural fruit sugars will cut down the temptation to go out and have a double chocolate malt. Cut the fruit into small pieces; drink fruit juice through a straw.

• When you watch TV at night, plan to do something else, too, like knit. If you know you will want to put something in your mouth, arm yourself ahead of time. Have a can of club soda or fruit juice and take a sip when you feel a nicotine fit coming on.

• Tell yourself throughout the day that just because you quit smoking does not mean that you will gain weight. Tell yourself that you are in control of your life, the cigarettes and candy and cakes are not.

• Breathe deeply. Smokers usually reach for a cigarette when they are tense; but it certainly isn't the nicotine that calms them down—it's the deep breathing. So, when you feel the tension rising, relax your shoulders, look off into the distance, and take three deep breaths. You'll feel calmer right away.

▲▲▲

Desire in the Afternoon

The afternoon is the toughest part of the day to stay on a diet. The postlunch and predinner time from 3 to 6 P.M. is when most dieters feel deprived. Blood sugar levels are dipping, your energy is sagging, depression is setting in. Plan ahead and make a snack a part of the afternoon— sunflower seeds (full of vitamins), an apple, half a banana.

▲▲▲

30 Psychological Adjustment

or, What Do I Do Now That I'm Here?

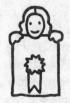

One day you will be thin. You will be so used to thinking of yourself as fat that it will actually catch you by surprise—in fact, everyone around you may notice it before you do. But suddenly—as if it all happened overnight—you will catch a glimpse of yourself in a mirror, perhaps when you are walking past a shop, and you will not recognize yourself. You will think "Who was that?" And then it will dawn on you that the person you didn't quite recognize right off the bat is the new you, the slim person you have always wanted to be.

Getting used to this new person is not necessarily going to be easy. Change, whether it be for good or bad, implies a disruption in the woof and warp of one's life, and until you settle into the new way, until it feels right, there will be moments of discomfort, of uneasiness, of being temporarily caught off guard. Count on them, and they won't get you down.

There is no way of telling exactly what is going to change in your life; all you can count on is that there will be change. People will respond to you differently, and you will find yourself reacting in ways that you never have before. Unless you are able to make the psychological adjustment that goes with the physiological change you have just come through, you will not wish to stay slim, for it will not feel comfortable. You may not be aware of what is going on or why you have started eating as you used to, but one day, there it will be, proof positive on the scales. We cannot tell you everything you should be prepared for; you will only know when the occasion arises how such and such is different from what has gone before. However, from the experiences of others and our own observations, here are some ideas to help you through the moments you may not have expected.

• Some people will resent you. Some of your acquaintances and friends, perhaps even your mate, have been quite comfortable in dealing, for better or for worse, with the old fat you. It was a kind of a deal you had struck up with them: I am a fat person; that is what I am like. Friends who stayed fat, others who have you in a notch that you no longer fit, may be at a loss as to how to deal with you. Some will not want to. Some will resent your being able to take control of your life when they cannot take control of theirs. You must go out of your way to reassure the people you care about that you value their love and friendship for exactly what it is: It is not a contract based on poundage. And the people who fall away from you, who do not really want reassurances or friendship with a new you, must be let go without guilt or remorse. Understand that their withdrawal does not mean you have turned into a bad person or an uncaring friend; it simply means that they don't know how, or don't want, to deal with the new you. All you can do is let them go gracefully; what you must not do is blame yourself.

• Your mate may have a particularly hard time. Some marriages are based on unspoken contracts: "I won't say anything about your eating, and you won't say anything about my drinking." And when the contract changes, the marriage may no longer work. You may want more, or something different, or someone different. If you want to make the marriage work, understand that your spouse is going through all kinds of worries and doubts about your new body image. "She's a knockout now—what will she want with me?" is not an uncommon reaction. A man who never had to worry about his wife at a party—surely the other men weren't going to be interested—now may be full of insecurities. "Who is that talking to her? They've been talking for a half hour! What's he trying to do?" The conversation may be as innocent as that of angels, and you will feel great because for the very first time in years you know that men find you attractive, yet when you try to tell your husband what a wonderful time you had, he interprets it quite differently from what you mean. He reads innuendo where it does not exist. A woman might think "Now that he's thin all the women will be after him—what will he want with me?" Reassure your mate frequently and with feeling. Even if it at first feels foolish to say the words, to give the extra loving pat, try to do it anyway because your mate needs to know that he or she continues to be needed and wanted. And be tolerant if your partner does or says things that do not seem quite reasonable.

• Beware of unrealistic fantasies. Years ago there was an advertising campaign based on how one could be the hit of any party if only one could sit down in front of a piano and play tunes while the rest of the gang sang along. Playing the piano might make some people the center of attention sometimes, but tickling the ivories certainly won't turn your life around. Losing weight is like that, too. Yes, it will change your life, but it will not turn you into the hit of the party or make you a superstar. If you couldn't dance before, or play tennis or ski, or whatever, you're not suddenly going to be able to do those things unless you take lessons. It is true that you will change as you grow thinner; you will learn new skills and improve others, but all that the actual weight loss will do is give you a sense of accomplishment and the confidence to branch out into other areas.

• Be aware that life as a slim person will not be one long roller coaster ride of unmitigated joy. If you didn't have a boyfriend before, then had one only for a month after you lost weight, don't despair. Lots of thin people have relationships that go *phfft!* after a week. Not every party will be fun and exciting; not every person of the opposite sex that you find appealing will respond in kind. Be prepared for a kind of letdown when the weight loss is over and your goal is reached. No one's life is without thorns among the roses. Don't despair or talk yourself back into eating because it wasn't worth it. "Why did I go to all that trouble if I can't have fun at every social gathering, if I can't find a mate by this time next week, if I don't get a better job in six weeks?" is a reaction that propels some people right back to the secret hot fudge sundaes. Don't give in. Perhaps the best plan is emotional self-defense: Expect to make gradual progress in new social and work situations, the same as you did with your weight loss—slowly, with peaks and valleys.

If you are going to try new experiences—like asking someone for a date—rehearse ahead of time. Start slowly. Instead of dinner and dancing at a fancy restaurant where you may be overwhelmed by the whole situation—try out your social skills in a more informal situation. A drink after work. A cup of coffee after class. A movie in the middle of the week. Bicycle riding in the park. Lunch. Plan what you are going to say. Write it out if you are really nervous. Talk it over with a close friend who has the social graces you desire, or with your therapist. And do not fall apart if you get turned down. The only way to find out if the excuse was real is to ask again. And again. Everybody has been turned down at one time or another. You have not been singled out by the gods. Try asking someone else. If you get turned down by a number of people, examine what might be wrong. Perhaps it is your manner, the type of activity you suggest, or maybe you are asking the wrong kinds of people. And when the affirmations start coming your way, go slowly. Rome and the new slim you weren't made in a day, and there's no reason to expect that you can learn to be socially proficient that quickly either.

• Don't misinterpret the words and actions of others. Okay, let's say that you're not a wallflower anymore; that a man comes up to you at a party, offers to get you another drink. That does not mean anything except that he wants to continue talking to you. It does not mean that he's only after one thing. Enjoy the flattery, but do not misread others' actions. A great number of women have worn their fatness as a protective shell for years, and when men are finally interested in them, they recoil in fear that they will be sexually used; it will only happen if you let it. In fact, you are more likely to be a target for such undesirable attention when you are fat, for some men will think: "She won't turn me down—she gets so few offers she'll be grateful."

• Be realistic. If someone talks to you, even asks for your phone number or says he would like to see you again, it does not mean he or she has fallen madly in love with you. Do not run out and hire the orchestra for the wedding. For the most part, people try to mean what they say. While thin people have practice at understanding the mating dance and its rituals, those who have been fat for years may have a hard time in the beginning. Overly romantic reactions to straightforward situations occur frequently among the formerly fat, but they can lead to unrealistic expectations and disappointments. On the other hand, don't doubt everyone or everything either. Something wonderful may indeed be happening. Eventually, you should be able to draw the fine line of distinction that separates illusion from reality.

• Don't give up what's nice about you. People who have some sort of physical cross to bear, whether it be an oversized proboscis or acne or fat, often develop certain sensibilities that make them quite wonderful people. They have used their wit, or their compassion, or their intellect, or charm to make up for what they saw as their lack. So now be grateful for the special qualities you know you possess; remember that every hardship teaches you to fall back on your inner resources, and has the potential to bring out the best in you, if you let it. So hang onto those acquired traits. A lot of people love you already for them.